T0195326

P. Van Den Heede
Osteopathic Medicine
Holonomic Keys for Treatment

To Sybille, my wife

To Elia, Iene, Jelle, and Simon, my children

Thanks to Jean-Pierre and Suzan for correcting the English vocabulary of the book

Patrick Van Den Heede

Osteopathic Medicine

Holonomic Keys for Treatment

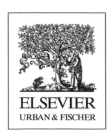
ELSEVIER
URBAN & FISCHER

URBAN & FISCHER München

All business correspondence should be made with:
Elsevier GmbH, Urban & Fischer Verlag, Lektorat Komplementärmedizin, Hackerbrücke 6, 80335 Munich, Germany, medizin@elsevier.com

Notice for the reader
The editors, authors and the publisher of this work have made every effort to ensure that the drug dosage schedules herein are accurate and in accord with the standards accepted at the time of publication. The reader is strongly advised, however, to check the product information sheet included in the package of each drug he or she plans to administer to be certain that changes have not been made in the recommended dose or in the contraindications for administration.

Bibliographic information published by the Deutsche Nationalbibliothek
The Deutsche Nationalbibliothek lists this publication in the Deutsche Nationalbibliografie; detailed bibliographic data are available in the Internet at http://www.d-nb.de/.

Content Strategist: Marko Schweizer, Munich/GER
Content Project Manager: Annekathrin Sichling, Munich/GER
Production Manager: Petra Laurer, Munich/GER
Formal Editor: Alfred J. Smuskiewicz, Lockport, Illinois/USA
Cooperative work: Jean-Pierre Lehr, Zwickau/GER
Illustrator: Martha Kosthorst, Borken/GER
Composed by: abavo GmbH, Buchloe/GER; TnQ, Chennai/IND
Printed and bound by: Printer Trento, Trento/I
Cover Illustration: Patrick Van Den Heede, Jelle Van den Heede, Orroir/BE; Martha Kosthorst, Borken/GER
Cover Design: SpieszDesign, Neu-Ulm/GER

ISBN Print: 978-0-7020-5263-7
ISBN e-Book: 978-0-7020-5264-4

Current information by **www.elsevier.de** and **www.elsevier.com**

Preface

Why do osteopaths describe biological facts in such mysterious ways? Terms such as "still point," "balance point," "listening" to the cranium, and "tissue memory" suggest a rather idiosyncratic descriptive approach to an anatomical and physiological domain that already has been described in detail by biomedical science. Perhaps one reason that osteopathy and biomedical science appear to have taken different paths is related to the osteopaths' rather philosophical approach to the body.

Nevertheless, the more I have studied and learned, the more I have become convinced that osteopathic philosophy and mainstream, or conventional, science could use the same nomenclature—because points of confluence do exist between their perspectives. In this text about tissue and the ways in which the osteopath can interact with it, I have tried to collect together histological, physiological, biochemical, and biophysical data to form a scientific substrate that can serve as a common frame of reference for both osteopaths and conventional biomedical practitioners and scientists. By examining a substantial amount of scientific outcomes in the field of tissue "behavior," I have become reassured and convinced that we osteopaths not only work in the same domain as the medical doctors, but also that many conventional scientific findings confirm the osteopathic methodology.

I suggest that we look at the relationship between the two fields from a different angle—perhaps it is the tissue and only the tissue that can serve to guide the two disciplines in the same direction of defining life. We should consider that osteopathy and biomedical science, each in its own way, is successfully explaining "what life means." The former is doing so through subtle touch; the latter by refinement of technological tools (eg, MRI, PET, ultrasound). I believe that quantum physics is an example of a science that has made great strides in this meaning-of-life adventure.

Results of any particular form of research are, in the end, defined only by the ways in which the research was conceived. Both osteopathy and conventional science are in search of the secrets of health. Sooner or later, for each research area being investigated by these disciplines, the outcome will be health itself. The tissue as a fundamental substance is the substrate upon which health is expressed and constantly reassessed. Studying this matter in its different modalities of expression will surely initiate us into the profound intimacy of life.

I have felt obligated to elucidate my "knowing" process for my students throughout Europe in order to help them in establishing useful directions for further research. Since 1986, I have taught at various colleges and given courses at numerous conferences throughout the continent, including Austria, Belgium, Finland, France, Germany, Italy, the Netherlands, Spain, and Switzerland. I have been honored that many students of osteopathy have been motivated to conduct their own research in areas related to my work. I hope this book will sustain, and even increase, their motivation while also carrying my perspective to a wider audience. In this regard, following are some relevant examples of students' theses that have been inspired by my work.

- Danjou J-L. Mobility/Motility of the Heart. Paris, France: French International Jury for Osteopathy; 1995.
- Dunshirn M. The Midline in Osteopathy. Vienna, Austria: Austrian International Jury for Osteopathy; 2006.
- Hunaut P. The Eye: Mirror of Man. Quebec, Canada: Canadian International Jury for Osteopathy; 1999.
- Jansen B. Influence of Osteopathic Manipulation on Secretion of Pancreas Polypeptides. Antwerp, Belgium: Belgian International Jury for Osteopathy; 1992.
- Langerotte A-M. Variations in Blood Parameters During Osteopathic Manipulation of the Ileo-cecal Region. Paris, France: French International Jury for Osteopathy, 1999.
- Lautenbacher T. Caecal or sigmoidal lift techniques by patients presenting a functional sciatic syndrome. Do these techniques have an influence on the degree of flexion of the leg during Lasègue test? Lausanne, Switzerland: Swiss International Jury for Osteopathy; ESO 2003/2004.

- Stelzer F. Accommodation Possibilities of the Eye and Possible Influence of Osteopathic Techniques on Presbyopia. Hamburg, Germany: German International Jury for Osteopathy; 2005.
- ten Ham EJ, et al. Strabism. Utrecht, Netherlands. Dutch National Jury for Osteopathy; 2004.
- Van Mechelen R. Influence of CV4 on Intra-ocular Pressure. Antwerp, Belgium: Belgian International Jury for Osteopathy; 1996.
- Villeneuve J. Harmonization of Heart Pulsation. Paris, France: French International Jury for Osteopathy; 1997.
- Voisard E. Osteopathy; Science and Wisdom. Paris, France: French International Jury for Osteopathy; 1990.
- Vuffray M. La Grande Manoeuvre Abdominale Hemodynamique. Lausanne, Switzerland: Swiss International Jury for Osteopathy; ESO 1999.
- Wyvekens M. Les Processus Moprhogéniques des Extrémités Supérieures pendant le Développement de l'Embryon Humain. Namur, Belgium: Jury National Belge d'Ostéopthie; 1991.

Patrick Van Den Heede, D.O.
Orroir (Belgium), July 2015

Acknowledgements

First of all, I would like to thank Jean-Pierre Lehr, DO, for patiently and carefully reading the manuscript for this book and for helping me eliminate unnecessary complexity in the text. Jean-Pierre is one of those "fundamentalist" osteopaths who continue to transmit the traditional osteopathic principles of A.T. Still. At his center Osteopathie im Hof in Zwickau, Germany, he and other renowned teachers work to convey these principles to younger practitioners, offering an excellent opportunity for less experienced osteopaths to gain familiarity with the fundamental aspects of this form of medicine.

It is clear that the kinds of teachings provided by Jean-Pierre support the continuity of the transmission of the most important message of the "old doc"—that osteopathy is an art of thinking about the origins of health and disease based on the elementary laws of the physiological integrity of all body mechanisms.

A second person I would like to thank is A.J. Smuskiewicz, for his constructive approach to editing the text for an American audience, as well as for his contributions to furthering the public understanding of osteopathy as a fundamental science about the knowledge of life.

Yet another individual I surely must not forget is Annekathrin Sichling, who helped immensely in interconnecting the various stages of the editing process and who provided the opportunity and means to get connected with the right persons to support this project.

I am also grateful to Sue Eveleigh, who helped to improve the text's readability together with Jean-Pierre.

Last but not least, I would like to thank Jelle, my daughter, for the wonderful illustrations that make the book much more attractive to read.

My sincere thanks to all!

Introductory considerations

It is apparent that the brain exerts a functional dominance over the rest of the body's physiological functions. The brain coordinates the vast majority of the neurological, neuro-endocrine, and immunological pathways. Although specific brain areas are concerned with pure reflex pathways and others integrate the more social, cognitive, or emotional aspects of being alive, it is certain that most of the entering and outgoing patterns pass through the central nuclei of the brain.

These central nuclei are integrated within the limbic-hypothalamic circuit, and they are dispatched to and from the cortex via the thalamic-reticular formation (ie, formatio reticularis) in ascending or descending pathways. The combinations of pathways form a "cluster of wires" that creates a diffuse patterning, though the pathways are able to organize well-defined interaction fields both within the brain and spreading from the brain to the periphery.

One has to remember that the brain, during phylogenetic and ontogenetic development, evolved as a centralized manager gathering and organizing peripheral information in various body patterns. It stored this information as functional units in different layers of its own organogenetic development. One can differentiate at least three evolutionary neuro-anatomical levels in the central nervous system (Fig. B.1). The first level belongs to the organization of the brain stem and the caudal mesencephalon, the second to the central nuclei organized around the thalamus, and the third to the peripheral cortex that evolved as a neocortical structure.

Most of the underlying functions are balanced via both sympathetic and parasympathetic tone within the autonomic nervous system. The balance is expressed between a "fear center" and a "pleasure center," which can be switched on or off in a decisive/nondecisive way. This is true not only for neurocognitive integration, but also for the neuroendocrine-immunological axis.

The cluster-of-wires concept elaborates on a forward- and backward-balancing mechanism of adaptability for the individual in regard to internal and external circumstances. The mean expression of all of these patterns can be perceived as a more or less functional state of homeostasis. The patterns of adaptation and reaction are partly determined genetically, though they are constantly adapting to the changing physiological needs of the individual. They represent a functional and dynamic memory that permits health to express itself.

Memory is believed to be a cortical function related to both conscious and subconscious states of interaction. In a certain way, memory is not only remembering, but also a process in which the body verifies the memory process—that is, the interactions in the body reinforce the conscious part of memory. At its most essential, memory is concerned with inherent patterns of adaptation through which the individual can adapt and make progress in life.

Much attention is given to the conscious part of memory—the part the individual masters by remembering and reproducing motor, cognitive, and emotional patterns of reaction and exchange. Most researchers have long agreed that memory is housed in the brain. In the past decade, however, a new approach, supported by scientific research, suggests that memory could be partially conditioned by tissue states. This concept means that the physiological state of a tissue (eg, the biochemical, biomechanical, or neuroimmunological state) could play a role in informing the brain about its functional level of vitality.

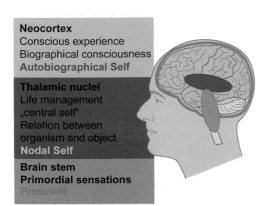

Neocortex
Conscious experience
Biographical consciousness
Autobiographical Self

Thalamic nuclei
Life management
„central self"
Relation between
organism and object
Nodal Self

Brain stem
Primordial sensations
Protoself

James Oschman[1] refers to such tissue as "the living, vibrating matrix." The extracellular matrix probably works by means of semiconduction in transmitting electrical coupling over long distances in the body. These semiconductive trains could reach the brain at a faster pace than even the fastest nerve conduction.

The tissue could represent a subconscious source of information that enters the brain, informing or directing the brain centers toward a less important level of consciousness and memory. Because the tissue works as a subconscious informer to influence the general state of brain activity, the conscious part of brain activity is probably the part that we can control and remember. However, the tissue also "adds" information to other body systems, such as the limbic system. This added interaction could be of supplementary—even directory—value to memory.

Thus, the nature and quality of activity displayed by the brain—conscious or subconscious—is partly determined by tissue activity and tissue tone. The memory patterns that can be released could depend on a summation of incoming information gathered from throughout the body, rather than an isolated function of a particular brain area. The tissue gives the signal; the brain then releases memory or triggers an adapted reaction pattern.

The "tissue state" or "tissue tonus" is partly transmitted to the brain by small-fiber pain receptors called alpha-receptors, which inform the brain via the lateral spinothalamic tract. They not only inform the somatosensorial area around the central sulcus, but the information is also sent to a deeper level of the frontal cortex—the insula. According to contemporary understandings, the somatosensory cortex localizes the information, while the deep cortex interprets it. The insula can be considered partly as a chemical interpretation center, where a variety of sensory inputs are interpreted to produce a mean value of our actual tissue state.

We could propose (or suppose) that the insula produces a map of our interoceptive body. It would thus be a functional part of our brain that frees and organizes function dependent upon an internal perception of tissue. Although it functions similarly to the rest of the brain, its source of information is quite unusual—namely "tissue state." This is called interoception, and this interoceptive cortex not only reacts to pain stimuli, but it also reacts upon subliminal stimuli in the physiological balanced field of the tissue. It is a system that receives information from the "tissue world" while integrating gustatory, olfactory, and auditory stimuli. The interoceptive cortex (ie, the cingulate-amygdala-insula-septal area) prepares the brain to function in an adaptive state of interactive awareness; this is one form of arousal. It is clear that the actual state of a tissue area is interpreted, and perhaps resolved, locally.

However, why couldn't it be possible that, under well-defined circumstances, the activity of tissues not only resolves an actual imbalance, but at the same time releases old energy accumulations—eventually activating memory centers in the brain via the interoceptive cortex?

We described the insula as an area filled with chemical receptors. Thus, it should not be surprising that any interaction with any tissue, anywhere in the body, is capable of releasing specific amounts or specific chemicals. The neuronal pathway, which is activated in this way, leads to the release of particular chemical and electrical impulses or reactions, which "train" the brain. This training means that one field with a specific wave-pattern (ie, frequency) is able to induce the function of another field. In other words, fields are able to influence other fields and to function together coherently, even at a distance. The interoception pathway appears to provide a possible mechanism for tissue normalization leading toward a physiologically balanced state that may modulate brain arousal.

It seems possible that physical components altered by such processes as inflammation, infection, or trauma also provide information to the brain when they enter during a state of biochemical and/or mechanical equilibrium. This process could be interpreted as the memorizing part of therapeutic normalization. It remains somewhat amazing that through the normalization of tissue, some patients are able to remember the precise circumstances that caused the restriction in the first place. For such a result to occur, the brain must, in addition to registering pain

---

[1] Oschman JL, Oschman NH. Somatic recall, part 1: soft tissue memory. Massage Ther J. 1995;34(3):36–45,66–67,101–167. Oschman JL. Trauma energetics. J Bodywork Movement Ther. 2006;10:21–34.

from the trauma, also store the content of the event in a time-related manner.

Accepting this point of view suggests that an important part of what we call memory is activated by tissue components. Touching the patient in the right place and at the right time can optimize the total integration of a therapeutic response. Touching the patient with "thinking fingers" certainly instructs the patient about a deeper dimension of physical awareness. Osteopathic treatments are not only about releasing restrictions, correcting imbalances, or bringing about a more homeostatic state. They also inform patients about their inner world—their tissue world. As R. Becker has said, "When you are on the body with both hands that are trustful and care for it, then the patient knows that something good is happening to him and he certainly will search for more."[2]

It is not because interoception[3] has been rediscovered and redefined that we can relate all memory as a reference of this tissue state. On the other hand, it is one of the most important ways by which the subconscious state of our tissue world reveals a part of its history.

Electrical fields in the body may be capable of polarizing and depolarizing effects in other parts of the body. It is possible that one of the largest electrical fields of our body—the brain—is constantly informed about these polarities. Besides the electrical fields, the fluids and the immune state of the body could also be considered as possible transmitters of information toward the brain.

Furthermore, the genetic, embryological, and developmental patterning of tissue, as well as other biochemical and biophysical events that could alter or inform the basic tissue state, are described elsewhere in this book. Hopefully, these discussions will give the reader a better understanding of the puzzle of this tissue world. The way in which the brain evolves during embryological and fetal phases is determined not only by genes (eg, Hox genes, pair-rule genes, segment polarity genes, gap genes, a multitude of morphogenes). Its morphogenetic patterning is as much influenced by environmental conditions, such

as the resistance of the developing cranium (ie, dural girdles), myelinization processes, and development of subsequent gyrations.

Much scientific study is currently being conducted on epigenetic factors that could alter or influence the patterning information behind the development of the brain. Such research suggests that the structuring of the brain's neural circuitry—in regard to programming and memory—is as much influenced by general morphogenetic parameters as by the specific genetic information for circuitry development. In addition to genetic controls, one could evoke molecular ordering and interactions, fluid pressure in the developing ventricles, electrical currents, and polarity development as cofactors for building brain structure and function.

Even in the adult brain (ie, full outgrown brain), a secondary, though less specific domain for integration of neural information could be established. Besides the neural circuits, there is a myelinated substrate enveloped by membranes that guarantees basic tonus (40 Hz) to the brain—the tonus by which it can program, integrate, and store information. Memory, as we know, is not stored in a specific place, but is the result of cooperative interaction between specific loci and larger brain areas. This fact implies that not all information exchanged between the brain and the rest of the body travels over neuronal pathways (eg, exteroceptive, interoceptive, proprioceptive). Rather, some parts of the information is "background noise" supplying the basic tonus of the brain.

These ideas, which are further explored throughout this book, offer explanations for the pathways and modalities by which the body articulates and connects the whole of its awareness and sensations to a higher center. It is, therefore, necessary to explore the lesser known domains of electrical, molecular, and fluid exchange of tissue to achieve a better understanding of the way the tissue communicates. Moreover, this discussion will help the reader understand that in the domain of consciousness and memory, there is not only one pathway from the body to the brain. Instead, there exists a complex network of pathways that function to coactivate the brain and the periphery and to support and evoke consciousness and memory.

The body participates actively in the support of consciousness, and the brain needs the body to feel the sources of its own comfort and discomfort. To search

2 Chila A. Course on fascial organization of the body. April 5, 2002; Namur, Belgium.
3 Willard F. Conference in Louvain La Neuve. April 2002; Belgium.

for the subtle interconnections between tissue and brain, or between tissue and heart, is one of the greatest tasks of the osteopath. This search is, in fact, the only way to understand the time/space relationship between the discomfort that is experienced by a patient and the real cause of that discomfort. It is the only clear path for the therapist to traverse in finding his or her way amidst the myriad of symptoms that are expressed.

The most valuable tools that the osteopath possesses are clinical skill and a deep knowledge about the entire array of interferences that can happen at the tissue level to determine the pathological program of the body.

Content

Picture credits

All drawings: Martha Kosthorst, Borken/GER

Figures 1.3, 2.2, 2.11, 2.17, 3.1, 3.2, 4.2, 4.6, 5.1, 5.2, 5.4, 5.5, 6.1, 6.2, 6.3, 6.4, 6.5, 6.8, 6.9, 7.1, 7.2, 7.4, 9.1, 9.2, 9.3, 9.4, Table 3.4a: Authorship drawing by Patrick Van Den Heede, Orroir/BE
Figures 2.3, 2.4, 2.5, 2.6, 2.7, 2.8, 2.9, 2.10, 2.12, 2.13, 4.5, 5.3a, 5.3b, 5.3c, 5.6: Authorship text by Patrick Van Den Heede, Orroir/BE; authorship drawing by Jelle Van Den Heede, Orroir/BE
Figures 2.14, 2.15, 2.16, 3.3, 3.4, 4.1 (left side), 4.3, 4.4, 7.3 (left side), 8.1, 8.2: Authorship text by Patrick Van Den Heede, Orroir/BE; authorship drawing by Patrick Van Den Heede and Jelle Van Den Heede, Orroir/BE
Figure 6.6: Patrick Van Den Heede and J-L Danjon. *Das kardiovaskuläre System in der Osteopathie.* Elsevier Urban und Fischer, München 2013

CHAPTER

1

Osteopathy and its interactions among different kinds of tissue organizations

1.1 Osteopathic interactions defined

It is accepted that osteopathic normalization achieves the following results:
- restores mobility of tissues and joints
- frees and enhances fluid exchange (ie, blood, lymph, extra– and intracellular fluid balance)
- normalizes neural, vegetative, and endocrine levels of interactions
- interferes positively with the immune system of the individual to establish basic homeostasis in every specialized function and form of the body.

We can assume that osteopathic normalization exerts its mechanical interference by acting through one particular, differentiated tissue-substance that relates all structures, forms, and functions at various levels and depths of the body. This tissue-substance is the mesoderm, together with one of its derivatives, the mesenchymal tissue. The properties of this tissue-substance and its cells are expressed in the following functions:
- linking tissue
- mechanical and biochemical exchange
- expressing direction, fixation, motility, mobility, and vibration (frequency)
- possessing tissue memory (eg, embryological, functional, and traumatic)
- influencing the biochemical environment of the whole body as a fundamental substance known as the extracellular matrix
- establishing a "whole body organ" that creates bodily dimension, rhythm, and time.

The mesenchymal tissue[1] transformations appear to be the most potent cell and tissue developments during embryo growth and through adult life, permitting adaptations to the alternating demands of structuring and functioning.

The different types of mesenchymal tissue are as follows:
- ectomesenchyme
- endomesenchyme
- mesomesenchyme.

The capabilities of the mesenchymal tissue can be used as a tool by the osteopath to interfere with all kinds of tissues and forms. It seems possible to enhance all types of function by manipulating this tissue through osteopathic techniques, including thrust technique, myotensive technique, fascial technique, myofascial unwinding, and reflex techniques.

The particular osteopathic intervention that is most effective appears to be dependent upon the degree of depth of the lesion. Such interventions are, therefore, applicable almost exclusively to functional states involved in the decrease of health and homeostasis. The tissue lesion cannot be in an irreversible condition, but only in a less pronounced state of deterioration of inner physiology, in the mechanical and biochemical sense.

The question remains whether an osteopath really knows what he or she is doing when manipulating a body structure. Is the osteopath correcting a dysfunction, liberating a blocked energy transformation, or informing a structure by restoring patterns of homeostasis? Alternatively, is he or she perhaps inducing a pattern the body cannot accept?

Another interesting question is whether the osteopath is restoring mobility or whether restored mobility is an expression of restored physiology? Could it be that mobility is only one of the expressions of altered physiology, and that the actual mechanism of restoring health involves restoring vital energy through liberation of specific tissue inhibitions—inhibitions that could have biomechanical, biophysical, or biochemical origins?

---

[1] Mesenchymal tissue has conjunction abilities; it is mobile, basophilic, and pluripotent; it undergoes many mitoses, and it builds 3-D networks.

1

Perhaps we have to reconsider what Still said about restoring the arterial nourishment of an organ or a tissue[2] to obtain a clearer understanding of the "drugstore" of the body.

The aim of an osteopath is not to manipulate just for the sake of manipulation, but rather to interfere with the loss of homeostasis of the body—a principle expressed very well in *The Respiratory and Circulatory Model of Gordon Zinc*, proposed by P. Masters. An osteopath must think about the disturbances that are exchanged between different body systems or tissue-organizations to validate a type of interference, rather than simply impose a strategy the body cannot accept. We would be wise to contemplate the idea expressed by Masters [1] during a conference: *"sooner or later osteopathy should become a cellular practice."*

1.2 Is mobility and/or loss of mobility the only tool in diagnosis and treatment?

Every tissue system has a typical pattern of mobility organization and mobility expression. This is true on a macroscopic as well as a microscopic level. Osteopaths claim that skilled hands can perceive both types of expressions.

The most evident expression of mobility is found in biomechanical studies, where axes and degrees of movement of joints can be precisely defined. If we concentrate on more hidden kinds of mobility and motility, then certainly the visceral and cranial fields are excellent domains of investigation.

The two most evident possibilities of research in the visceral domain have been:
- mobility and/or loss of mobility of an organ, as in physiology, a-physiology, and pathology
- the study of structure and function as functional units sustaining the equilibrium of a particular physiological system (eg, digestion-metabolism).

Questions that should interest every osteopath in search for causality in pathological expressions of physiology are the following:

From the osteopathic point of view, which is the missing link between function, loss of function, and pathology—in contrast to the classical medical approach to the problem (eg, virology, traumatology, hematology)? Furthermore, which substrate, other than that found and studied in classical medicine, could be causal in inducing pathology? We could also ask ourselves about the type of tissue in which physiological and pathological events take place.

When we eliminate each element that could create a particular symptomatology (eg, virus, bacteria, ischemia, compression, tumor), we could detect one specific tissue function and interaction organizing every physiological and a-physiological event and condition. Apparently all function and transformation is based upon basal mesenchymal-epithelial exchange, a process that starts early in embryogenesis. This type of exchange is possibly one of the earliest primary reactions of cells in tissue construction and metabolism. Could it also be true that the net result of every type of manipulation (eg, touch, incision, injection) induces changes in tissue behavior through this type of interaction?

It was E. Blechschmidt [2] in one of his books about his research on embryos, who stated that form, structure, and topography were three essential factors to create what he called biodynamic construction-movements. In his opinion, these biodynamic movements were organized by molecular and submicroscopic matter movements conceived for abolishing regional tissue resistances. In this way, these exchanges can be conceived as early physical performances.

An osteopath could imagine that what Blechschmidt calls "enhancing mobility, freeing mobility" is perhaps sustained and effective only by this primitive tissue reaction. This would mean that the osteopath is not enhancing mobility as much as enhancing tissue interaction, which, in its own way, is enhancing the improvement of mobility. In this sense, mobility becomes a "way" rather than a "tool" to express tissue integrity.

An osteopath should know that his or her focus is defined by tissue expressions as well as mobility, rather than exclusively by mobility. Of course,

---

2 "the law of artery is supreme"

mobility is an interesting subject for research, serving as an academic reference indicating improvement or impairment of function. However, a better area of investigation could be whether mobility sustains physiology or instead is a part of physiology. In other words, is mobility determining or determined by physiology? If it is determining physiology, then we should ask about its specific interaction and place within physiology. Isn't mobility—which is firstly a molecular, electrolytic event—processing on the level of tissue and sustaining more macroscopic events than mechanical events? A rhetorical question could be: is the outcome of mobility *moving* or *exchanging?*

We can assure ourselves that classical medicine has also studied the mobility of organs. We know that the kidneys, the pancreas, and also the heart all possess a degree of mobility that can be measured efficiently by scientific tools. [3–16]

The osteopath can be satisfied that the viscera are mobile, and their degree of mobility can be quantified. For most of us, it has been the discovery of the 20th century. However, other questions are probably more urgent for this 21st century.

Does mobility support a specific type of physiology, or is it an integrating part of all physiology? Can mobility be a quantifying element in evaluating digestive, urogenital, or cardiopulmonary physiology? If so, how can mobility and this particular aspect of physiology, which is the common substrate that participates in both functions (motion and specific function), be correlated?

Is tissue integrity an important topic to be studied in the near future? We have seen tissue integrity explored in such domains as the "tensegrity" concept.[3] [17] In this concept, the metabolic and mechanical functions are integrated in one and the same

domain—at the level of biomolecular exchange. D. Ingber, in one of his numerous articles, writes that the whole cytoskeleton of the cell functions as a tensegrity system that can influence even the nucleus and its DNA transcription modalities.

Could it be that the medical doctor and the osteopath have to study the same substrate to justify the results of their therapeutic measures? Perhaps the biomolecular (ie, cellular) level is "the common place" for both doctor and osteopath. Perhaps this infinite little cell contains the secret of all interactions.

One particular tissue is the quintessence of these epithelial-mesenchymal exchanges—the mesenchyme and the extracellular matrix, as described by Pischinger. [18]

1.3 The major organizer of mobility

We generally agree that there are two types of mobility: a microscopic tissue motility and a macroscopic, mechanical mobility.

Tissue mobility is based on:
- electrophysiological exchange
- nourishing metabolic currents, dependent on such measurable factors as:
  - "space" that creates the possibility for currents to exhibit exchange
  - heat gradients that sustain exchange of metabolites
  - electrical potentials
- extinction of currents dependent upon cell apoptosis.

These were the "laws" as stated by E. Blechschmidt [19] in his work on biodynamics in embryology. If we accept the statements of Blechschmidt, we could postulate that during tissue organization, genetic and epigenetic factors interfere. The sum of these interferences creates a preference for cell maturation, differentiation, and orientation. Cells are orientated in a virtual body plan in which they migrate and use environmental influences to develop their provisional or definite function.

---

3 In a study on brain plasticity after birth, it was shown that in visual cortex neurons, the enzymatic activation of c-AMP by adenyl-cyclase is the first step in intracellular protein folding, changing their three-dimensional pattern and, thereby, their biological activity. It is clear that the activated protein kinases, by phosphorylation and dephosphorylation of certain proteins, determine major aspects of neuron activity, including their fluctuating changes in shape and the intracellular traffic of molecules between dendrites and the cell body. The neuron specific protein MAP2 (microtubule-associated protein) plays an important role in modulating the biochemical and mechanical pattern of the neuron.

Besides the genetic patterning that organizes a great deal of the future body axles and cell/tissue induction, differentiation, and specification programs, there are also physical factors that interfere to create a useful biodynamical interference field. This field, for a major part, is responsible for creating the epigenetic landscape for morphogenetic processes.

Progression of cells in their spatial environment is sustained by the following three factors:

- tension, organized by transmembraneous electrolyte exchange
- heat, produced by metabolite exchange and organized by the bloodstream
- vacuum/hypotension, organized by cell death and pressure differences.

In this way, blood vessels, membranes, and fascial tissue build an important frame for the structure and form of the developing anatomical entities. They also display a possible memory framework on which other motions are based. Part of tissue memory lies in this collagen, elastin, and fibrin network that contains the "microtimes" of genesis and actualized function.

Mechanical mobility can be defined as the result of these microscopic movements, which take place during subsequent phases of developmental biology. In fact, it is a reality that most of the organs expressing a proper mobility received this mobility through three major developments that organized the spatial environment of the body during embryology: hepatization, cardialization, and cerebralization. The final mobility and motility of each organ is organized and guided by these previous paths of spatial organization in the body.

Mobility is made possible by specific tissue developments supporting the needs of functional and spatial organization of the respective sequences of development, as discussed in the following three points.

1.3.1 Tissue and cell-environment interaction

Tissue organization is based on ecto-mesenchymal or epithelial-mesenchymal interactions and transitions. Two different cell populations play a role in further specification of function and interactions:

the neural crest cell lineage and the undifferentiated mesenchymal cell lineage. Both populations display not only specific functions on the moment of their differentiation, but also show an adaptive behavior dependent upon environmental needs and information.

These cells organize the major portion of the mechanical potential of tissue. Although they can be found at many levels in the body, they retain in their cell memory as part of their original information and time induction. This means that they probably continue to be linked in their actual function by the time and tissue pattern by which they originally started their differentiation. We can define this as "inductive synchronicity," [20] a term meaning that different tissue origins are organized and programmed at the same time during their development.

This fact also creates the probability that tissue dysfunction in a particular part of the body could disturb tissue interaction in a completely different part of the same body, which is possibly expressed in other parts of physiology. Loss of mobility can originate in the dysfunction of a tissue that at first glance displays no functional link with the changes that were found.

1.3.2 Tissue and genetic factors

Besides the cell-environment interaction, a second interference is important. A large portion of cell function is genetically determined by information that depends on homeobox genes, qualifying the organization and segmentation of interaction on different tissue levels.

Early in embryological development (fourth week), rhombomeres are formed as the result of mechanical interference of the growing neurectoderm upon its nearest environment—the stomodeal membrane and the underlying endoderm. The rapidly growing brain becomes larger and heavier than what could normally be sustained by tissue. That is why the tissue interferes in a mechanical way upon its own form. A bending forward process is initiated, and both brain and primitive foregut undergo typical patterns of spatial organization, partly initiated by homeobox genes and partly dependent on environmental interference (➤ Fig. 1.1).

The developing mesoderm, lying between both protagonists, is induced at almost the same time and exhibits a typical pattern of somitomere formation preceding the definitive somite formation. It progresses in a typical frequency of 7 somitomeres lying ahead of the inductive notochord and 11 somitomeres lying behind the somite that had been formed before (➤ Fig. 1.2). Both occurrences result in the

further topographical organization and migration of the neural crest cells, necessary for informing, establishing function, and linking spatially separated tissues. This link can be expressed in different properties of the informed tissue, as we can read in the works by Carlson. [21]

The neuro-endocrine and vascular routes seem to be elected pathways by which anatomical barriers

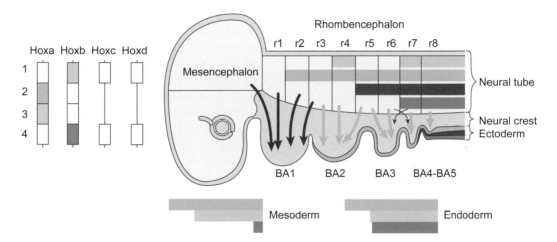

Fig. 1.1 Anterior to posterior polarizing by Hox genes at the level of rhombomere 2

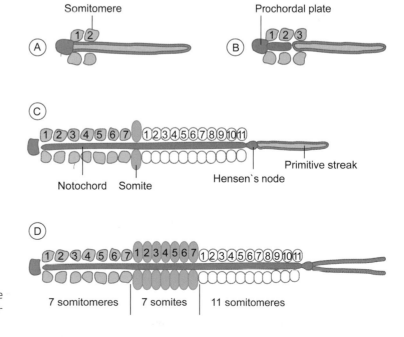

Fig. 1.2 Regression of primitive streak and simultaneous maturation of somitomeres into somites

are transgressed or organized. (As A.T. Still mentioned in *The Philosophy and Mechanical Principles of Osteopathy,* "the law of artery is supreme.")

1.3.3 Tissue and integrative pattern

A third property of tissue has to be considered. Tissue is not only linked with other tissues by typical cell-cell interactions, cell-environment interactions, and genetically defined patterns of segmentation and distribution of function. There is also the property of the conjunctive tissue, which Pischinger [22] called "the fundamental substance."This means that tissue can build its own integrative pattern in a strictly local reaction, or it can elaborate a more complex reactive pattern irradiating over the whole body. Both possibilities exist because each part of tissue is linked to specific reactive agents in loco (fibroblasts, capillary network, nerve terminals), and it is also linked to more integrative poles in the body—just as there are the reticulo-endothelial, hormonal, and neural poles. The net result is that a local tissue disturbance tends to be resolved at the place of the preferred conflict. If not resolved, the disturbance could interfere with more general patterns of integration in the different enumerated poles.

Therefore, Pischinger states that the summation of stimuli can alter or determine the total body tonus in a more sympathetic or parasympathetic reaction pattern. The local disturbance can be understood as a tissue "cyst," organized by a "lymphoid-plasmatic" plaque [23], a kind of depolarized cell cluster that inhibits surrounding reaction units of cellular organization.

The functional state of the body is dependent on a more local or a more general state of toxicity of the tissue (ie, disturbance of the cell redox system). Physical interference with the tissue by means of needle stimulation, or infiltration with xylocaine or procaine, could balance the inhibited physiology into a more functional pattern.

1.3.4 Tissue in osteopathy

Osteopathy—through its mechanical interference with the tissue—can perhaps do more than only restoring mobility. Possibly, an aimed interference with soft tissue enhances the self-healing function of the body by eliminating tissue cysts, rather than restoring pure mobility. We can suggest that enhancing a cell-to-cell interference in the whole array of physiological expressions may also enhance mobility in a more general way.

In conclusion, we can suggest that at least three tissue properties participate in conditioning the reactive environment of the body:

• the epithelial-mesenchymal cell-to-cell interactions

• the conditioning effect of the pattern formation by gene information

• the connective tissue, acting as a fundamental substance to integrate cell-cell reactive patterns and more generalized patterns of the whole body.

The union of these three agents creates, as Ader [24] described in 1981, the psycho-neuro-immunological environment that interferes with all bodily functions—as the mechanical, digestive, neurological, endocrine, and immune systems express them.

For the osteopath, this means that it is possible to interfere, by way of a rather mechanical approach to the body, with all of these specific functions at the same time. The integrative capacity of the body can restore function in every part of the body in an appropriate proportion through only one stimulus or only a few stimuli. [25]

Perhaps this also means that restored mobility is a qualitative factor indicating enhanced digestion or immune function. It is also possible that the different degrees of mobility, which indicate a loss or gain in motion, are much more important as reliable indicators of gain and loss of function in the associated tissue on different levels, as previously enumerated. Another consequence is that tissue is the main processor integrating all the other physiological patterns and, thus, also the main tool for normalization of these functions.

An example could help explain this better: As long as a certain trigger point exists somewhere in a tissue (eg, a focal infection of a tooth), it will be impossible to normalize the neurological tension of the body. Once the trigger point is liberated, the neurological tension will be restored automatically, or with only slight help from the osteopath.

An osteopath interferes with the body by way of enhancing tissue exchange, which supports the basic components of homeostasis in a biological system:
- support of energetic supply of the cell-metabolism
- support of osmotic and oncotic forces necessary for exchange
- support of hydrostatic and hemodynamic forces necessary for exchange, posture, and movement.
- support of gaseous exchange necessary for stability of pressure gradients in blood and lungs.

1.4 Tissue and cells as a mechanical integrative system

Every physical system that is subjected to the laws of gravity and motion displays a well-defined structure that permits interaction, integration, and translation of chemical and mechanical impulses. Every impulse, as minimal as it is, can be considered as a message for the modeling of reaction patterns of the body.

Physical structures are built up in geometric triangular, pentagonal, or hexagonal patterns that integrate mechanical stresses by mechanical traction or compression impulses. Rigid tubes that become compressed can eventually exert a traction force upon elastic elements from the same or adjacent microstructures, which are involved in the same process. Stability of a mechanical system is warranted in the way that an increase in tension will be equilibrated by an increase in compression.

Cells and tissues can be considered in the same manner—especially because cells display a particular specialized mechanical integration system built up by the cytoskeleton of the cell. [26] Microfilaments, intermediary filaments, and microtubules construct this cytoskeleton. The nucleus also possesses the same microfilaments, which are in direct mechanical contact with the DNA and RNA material of the cell. Moreover, these same cells are linked to the extracellular matrix by mechanical linking proteins, known as integrines.

It is generally accepted that changes in form and movement of cells are the result of modulation of

tension or chemical remodeling. We can conclude that the architecture and chemical composition of a tissue unit are dependent upon these same two processes.

This interference was defined as a tension-integration pattern called tensegrity. [27–35]

The action pattern of tensegrity is based on the degree of prestrain in a given tissue. Cells of this tissue are capable of creating harmonious vibrations that translate a mechanical-chemical energy by the way of waving movements. The integrines serve as mechanoreceptors. They can activate or inhibit the transmission of the expressed force to the extracellular matrix or to the cytoskeleton.

This exchange is, in fact, bidirectional, and the transmission is effectuated by molecular modulation. A local signal can evoke global response of the whole body. According to the law of linear stiffening, if the degree of prestress increases, this response is transferred to the whole pattern of the body.

As a provisional conclusion, we could suggest the following:
- The degree of mechanical action seems to correlate well with an increase of metabolic activity in the same cell compartment.
- There exists simultaneously an ubiquity of transmission of the mechanical signal in the totality of the body.

These observations should inspire the osteopath in deepening his or her concept of mechanical interaction with the body. In this way, a better understanding of the whole body can be achieved.[4]

1.5 What is tissue memory, and which factors contribute to it?

Memory appears to be one of the major organizers of the functioning of the body. Part of memory is an integrated form of adaptation to environmental factors obtained through the ontogenetical, and

---

[4] Zink JG, Lawson WB. An osteopathic structural examination and functional interpretation of the soma. *Osteopath Ann.* 1979;7:12–19.

perhaps the phylogenetical, necessities of coping with changing environmental information. This means that all structure is at the same time an end result of ontogenetical and phylogenetical patterning. In addition, it is also a possibility for new adaptive integration of all kinds of stresses (eg, mechanical parameters as well as chemical-molecular reactions).

One view of the genetic database, as suggested by Chauvet [36] is that it is nothing more than a reproduction of effective, temporary adaptations to environment. Memory is acquired information that is probably stocked in every constituent of the body. Anatomy is memory, physiology is memory, and biochemistry is memory. The only difference between these three enumerated participants of organizing interaction with the environment is that there is a certain aspect of complexity in their construction that interferes with their definitive function.

We have to consider that each tissue has its own complexity, acquired by developmental and functional cues. In this way, each tissue can express a different part of a time/space relationship, which we are searching for.

From this perspective, anatomy seems to encompass older information than the adaptive functions of physiology or the integrative and transforming functions of biochemistry. This is why adaptation is not only an expression of function but also of time— because it is related to different moments of adaptation throughout phylogenetic and ontogenetic events.

A second characteristic of memory is that it expresses a certain depth. It includes all the different physiological and hierarchical levels of tissue organization, ranging from molecular to cellular to tissue to organ. A wide variety of compounds, ranging from cell adhesion molecules to growth factors or mechanical organizers, are involved in building this particular part of our memory. Specific types of such compounds include proteoglycans, glucosaminoglycans, collagen, and fibrin.

Space is another constructive field where function is related to an integrated and adaptive memory. We need a structure to express function as part of our integrative, adaptive, or expressive capability. The soundest and most extensive study conducted about space-time relationship in humans is the research in the embryological domain.

Apart from other researchers, Chauvet[5] has succeeded in defining specific space-time relations relating function to tissue organization or maturation. A remarkable fact is that Chauvet did not continue this research throughout the complete human life span. He partially described the major events of infancy. However, according to his observations, as humans grow older, "the less specific the space-time schedules are defined."

There are two possible explanations for these observations:

- Perhaps Chauvet did not recognize the continuity of cellular and tissue transformation through the entire lifespan and concentrated too much on cell and tissue disintegration. As a result, he became entangled in a never-ending search for pathological events.
- Alternatively, as humans develop, we become increasingly liberated from the old constructions and patterns. In this way, we build more flexible forms of adaptation to the environment and also a more personalized form of functioning. The more we age, the more we become specialized in interacting with and modulating our environment.

Part of this saved ontogenetic information is used as the basic substrate for function. However, through earlier development and maturity, tissue can either omit or lose basic transformations for adapting better to new physiological strategies. Nevertheless, we should not forget that human life continues to be a specialized attempt at finding adaptations to self-induced disturbances of both Mother Nature and perhaps also our own nature. This means that the old patterns of structure/function relationships are progressively transformed into more adapted patterns, which we could interpret as more specialized.

- Humans are the only creatures capable of disrupting their own environment so profoundly that

---

5 "A physical system is not in evolution by self-reproductive processes; it cannot accumulate the selective advantages of regulatory cycles obtained during evolutionary episodes. A biological system, on the other hand possesses an astonishing array of complex functional interrelations guarantying homeostasis of this open system." Cfr. Chauvet G. pp. 98-99.

they might fail, ultimately, to adapt to changes that they have made around themselves. We are perfectly capable of destroying our own environment.

From these realizations, two provisional conclusions can be proposed:

- Human life is, in part, a continuation of the "hierarchic system building" that occurs during embryological differentiation and, thus, a continuing attempt at adaptation.
- Therapy could concentrate on counteracting pathological differentiation of cells and tissues, or it could focus on sustaining further cell and tissue adaptation to continuous environmental changes. The first form of therapy is curative, the second preventative.

Returning to the subject of memory, we are obliged to make a distinction between the conventional term and a more expansive, more useful definition of memory.

- In general, we can postulate that there exists a genetic memory, of which certain "mutations" are attempts at adaptation to environmental changes. From this perspective, the genetic material seems stable, though certain expressions display instability.
- The immune system can be considered a second form of memory. The typical patterns of immune reactions (type I, II, III, IV) have a certain degree of predictability and relate the present state of the organism to its past.
- A third pattern is the cognitive memory, through which we can store patterns of concepts in a specialized tissue—the brain. This tissue, we believe, integrates all possible functions, including motor, intellectual, psychological, affective, and emotional. It is important to remember that every memory requires simple tissue reaction patterns (such as those involving O^2-consumption and glycogen) for their energetic needs. Certainly, humans can memorize very complicated formulas and sentence structures. But is this not possible while there is some freedom in tissue adaptation?

This question can be considered quite simply, by considering other, similar questions. When your belly is aching, do you still possess the same capability of using your brain as when your belly feels fine? Is it not true that when your body is focused on the more urgent needs of coping with pain and trying to restore a certain degree of homeostasis that it is difficult to delve into the depths of your conscious memory? Does it (the consciousness of the body) not claim deeper forms of organization than pure cognitive processes? Does this not prove that there exists depths of functioning that support more superficial, free forms of behaving? In other words, the more there is an urge for survival, the more the cognitive part of consciousness will be controlled by archaic patterns belonging to the limbic system.

Perhaps the deeper we go in tissue organization, the deeper we go in memory. Perhaps the brain is only the software of deeper-layered memories that can be actualized by "pure" tissue experience. [37]

As stated in the work of Blechschmidt and Gasser [19], the primary motor information to the brain is an afferent "fluxion" (a metabolic flux), capable of organizing the motor areas of the developing brain. In this concept, the brain is only stocking peripheral information from important tissues during a particular period of their development (eg, the hands folded around the heart bulge.) Blechschmidt states that tissue in its autonomous functioning is the primary source of brain development, even before a neurological afference exists. Fluxion is the term he uses for the afferent pathways to the brain that transmit this kind of tissue information.

Perhaps the brain provides us with the possibility of linking old memories to newer forms of interaction with the environment. The brain can go back and go forward on the condition that tissue does not make a repetition. When tissue is free, the cognitive memory can link past and future. Otherwise, it transcribes past in the future under the form of subconscious levels of interaction. In this way, part of our freedom is determined by the past—perhaps by old tissue structures (eg, reflex patterns).

Even when osteopathic treatment has succeeded in relieving a major part of a patient's symptoms, we still must ask whether a remnant of the problem remains hidden in the body's structure as information that could eventually lead to a new pattern of symptoms. This can be answered only by paying attention to the tissue and the varying degrees of density of its organization. Different densities reflect different levels of restrictions in physiological exchange. These are expressed by different parameters, such as heat, fibrosis, loss of mobility, and depth of tissue restriction. These memories express themselves in different forms that permeate as more severe or less severe pathological alterations in tissue.

We can look at the presence of microbes as both indicators and organizers of altered states of tissue health. *Staphylococcus aureus*, for example, can be found in both pulmonary tissue. leading to pneumonia, or in an osseous part of the body, creating osteomyelitis. It is clear that this bacterium can hide itself for a long time, creating a home base from which it organizes only transient febrile periods. However, the bacterium could also cause profound alterations in distant joints to create an arthritic pattern of body functioning.

From a functional medical or naturopathic perspective, it is apparent that even when a germ has been considered to have been eradicated, it can still hide as a less virulent form and "awaken" several years later in response to a change in the weather or even an intense emotional experience. One example of these concepts are the "focal infections" in the roots of teeth that are seen by both neural therapists and homeopaths as major causes of disease, especially of the joints and digestive tract. Carlson [21] provides us with similar information when dealing with the maturation of the different neurite growth cones.

The properties of most of the molecules involved in inflammatory patterns (eg, cytokines, endotoxins, enzymes) exist to increase the toxemic state of the body and to involve distant body systems in the same reaction pattern. On the level of the extracellular matrix, Pischinger [13] mentioned the existence of "lympho-plasmatic plaques" as capable of local interference, blocking local physiological tissue exchange. To the greatest possible extent, these processes could disturb the organization of the whole body.

In a certain way, we could ask ourselves if a simple fibrosis formed by scar tissue or as a remnant of direct trauma could not organize a major part of the memory of the organism without impinging in any apparent way on the conscious or subconscious level of the brain. We could look at certain autoimmune diseases (such as neurofibromatosis or lupus erythematosus) as expressing this fibrosis in a different way. The state of tissue could be altered by long-lasting

infectious or inflammatory processes, triggering a cascade of autoimmune reactions that specifically aggress certain kinds of tissue. Perhaps the tissues express only another depth and time dimension of fibrosis, or perhaps they display another dimension of acquired memory.

Based on this concept, even a twisted ankle could be capable of altering body proprioception and even interfering with memory by creating local fibrous tissue. One of the most fascinating structures on the biochemical level of tissue functioning may be what Chauvet calls the "enzyme-substrate," which permits considerable acceleration of the body's biochemical reactions. We could see the interaction between an enzyme and its particular substrate as one of the earliest memories of the body. The enzyme cannot only react on its specific target molecules, but it also participates in triggering inflammatory processes in tissues distant from its site of action.

There are two ways to interfere with a chemical enzymatic reaction.[6] One way is to control the quantity of enzyme; the other is to change the structure of the enzyme. In the latter case, after alteration of the geometric

structure of the enzyme, the enzyme induces a structural modification of the cell substance. This type of enzyme regulation is called allosteric regulation. Enzymes catalyze every chemical reaction in a cell. Even genes require enzymes to affect their functions and changes.

Digestive enzymes, secreted by the pancreas, seem not only to be useful for aiding digestion, but some of the activated enzymes seem to be reabsorbed into the bloodstream to circulate in inactivated forms. These inactivated enzymes participate in local inflammatory processes far away from their site of secretion. Some authors define this processing as an "entero-pancreatic" cycle. [38]

We could suggest that, at its most basic, memory is probably dependent upon enzymatic processing at

---

6 "Deux mécanismes très sophistiqués paraissent être à la base de la chimie des systèmes vivants: l'interaction allostérique et la catalyse enzymatique." (Two very sophisticated mechanisms appear to be basic in biochemistry; the allosteric interaction and the enzymatic catalysis.) Cfr. Chauvet G. pp. 69-70.

a cellular and molecular level, while at the next level, geometric structural changes play a major role in signal translation and restructuring. The main function of the enzymes is to catalyze biomolecular reactions, including the synthesis of other proteins. The catabolic ability of enzymes depends crucially on their three-dimensional structure, which, in turn, depends on their L-amino acid sequence (enantiomeric configuration).

Enzymes seem capable of simultaneously modifying the biochemistry, the shape, and the function of a cell, as well as the proteins participating in the biomechanical pattern of the cell and cellular environment. This is the plasticity previously defined as tensegrity. Part of the memory seems cellular; part seems supported by geometric changes of participating chemical compounds. This also means that memory is possibly stored in the "silent compartments" of the body that, if stimulated, enhance conscious remembering by the brain through images or words.

M. Proust[7] once noticed that the simple smell of a particular type of cookie helped him to remember a specific experience of his youth. Thus, we could state that the physical fact of smell can evoke a particular information stocked in the subconscious. We could ask ourselves how much of the memories stored in our subconscious are sustained by stimuli we do not even notice, such as touch, smell, vision[8] and sound. [17]

Inversely, how much of the conscious information is stored in two compartments—partly in the brain and partly in a particular tissue? Both compartments can undergo a synchronous shock elicited by autonomic, vascular, or endocrine short-circuiting. This short-circuiting can function as a new mode of patterning for subsequent adaptive reaction modalities. As early as the 1930's, Kahn[9] wrote about the shock the body undergoes with sudden atmospheric changes or cold attacks, including how it undergoes an electrical short-circuit, paralyzing the autonomic exchange.

Apparently, the tissue is the first to integrate unacceptable information, and it probably also is the trigger that alters autonomic tonus, in the way Pischinger described in his books.

1.6 New principles in the structure-function relationships

The body, like all biological systems, strives for a certain hierarchical organization that permits it to function in an economically adapted pattern, in a way that guarantees velocity and precision. The current view is that, to a very important degree, speed of action and reaction is governed by the central nervous system, which integrates peripheral reflex patterns. Most manual therapists consider this system as the go between that integrates the signal of a manipulative act with the reaction of the tissue upon which the impulse was focused. Most often, the primary objective of treatment is to normalize the neurological or vegetative tonus of this system, through modulation by a so-called reflex arc.

The structure interfering with a system, as opposed to with one particular function, is another reaction pattern. The structure could be a spatial "physical" arrangement of elements of the system. [26] This system strives for stability, making its adaptation throughout different episodes of dissipating energy and then returning to physiological balance. These processes are accompanied by entropic and negentropic modes of energy management that correlate with the laws of conservation of energy, as defined in the thermodynamic laws of living systems. We can conclude that a structure always tries to return to its position of functional stability, using dissipating systems and energy conserving procedures.

---

7 Proust M. A la recherche du temps perdu.
8 In the so called "critical period" of brain plasticity after birth, the visual signal of light is decisive for the building of visual pathways and for activation of visual cortex neurons by actions of typical intracellular proteins, MAP2. The system of memorization seems to be hidden in a long chain of enzymatic interactions ranging from adenyl cyclase over c AMP to activating protein kinases and enhancing phosphorylation and dephosphorylation of certain proteins that are capable of determining the biochemical and biomechanical pattern of cells and cell environments.

---

9 Kahn F. Ton corps et toi. New York, 1939:256-266.

Through these procedures, it displays movements toward a point of balanced energy exchange, avoiding a definitive state of energy loss defined as thermodynamic equilibrium. A system can also integrate factors of different origin, which activate the same function.

The following example illustrates the complexity of interference in a physiological system.

The bulbar respiratory center is influenced by mechanical signals elicited in the lung alveoli and bronchioles, all integrated in the Hering-Breuer reflex. However, the same oscillatory respiratory neurons are also influenced by hydrogen ions in the cerebrospinal fluid bathing these respiratory neurons in the floor of the fourth ventricle. Furthermore, these same neurons respond to the oxygenation levels of hemoglobin, which can also produce an effect on respiration. Thus, we can see that what is apparently one neurological function is actually influenced by at least three different factors.

This "multitasking" is also evident in the cardiovascular system, which regulates blood pressure while simultaneously serving as a vector for endocrine molecules, as in transporting insulin to each cell in metabolic need. Does it so astonish, then, that a fall in blood sugar level is usually accompanied by changes in blood pressure? The hydrostatic force of cardiac pulsation and peripheral after-load is an important tool in sustaining the metabolic potency of the body. Apparently, both are functionally interrelated by subtle cellular impulses that also can destabilize the autonomic tonus of the body.

It is becoming increasingly evident that the body is not merely functioning through the connections of the well-defined anatomical pathways, as there are also other neurological reflex arcs and endocrine pathways. A most intriguing thesis is that the body is simultaneously functioning in several areas, each one capable of acting either as a "source" or as a "pit." Every area can have an emitting function related to a distant area, but it can also function as a receiver for other emitting areas. [36]

Osteopaths and even physical doctors should be aware of the fact that the body is not functioning merely in so-called linear patterns supported by anatomical and physiological relationships. Rather, a great part of interferences happens through field interactions. These field interactions are organized by a multitude of physical and chemical parameters that, when disturbed, can interfere with the integrity of another field. The parameters that organize the interactions between different fields include biochemical, biomechanical, chemo-electric, electrophysical, and electromagnetic components.

The functional go-between likely has to be sought in the functionality of the cell cytoskeleton and in the properties the extracellular matrix.

• The living matrix is composed of extracellular matrix and extracellular fluids, and it functions as a living substance that displays vibratory and electrical properties (cfr. J. Oschman. Vide supra).
• The cell cytoskeleton is specifically constructed to translate mechanical signals outside the cell in specific enzymatic, biochemical, and genetic translations.

As P.A. Janmey has written: *"A primary signal to many cell types is mechanical. Senses of hearing and touch are initiated by forces rather than molecules impinging on the cell surface that are later translated to the biochemical reactions leading to acute cellular responses. In addition, acute or sustained application of forces such as the shear stress produced by vascular fluid flow often leads to remodeling of cell morphology or to expression of specific genes. … However, for mechanical transmission to the cell interior, a three-dimensional elastic structure is required. In all these cases, signaling depends on elastic coupling between the site where the forces are applied and the potentially distant point at which the first biochemical change occurs."* [26]

Basically we are confronted with a subtle cell-signaling mechanism, described as tensegrity, and a multitude of functions that have to be integrated on this cellular level by way of mechanical transmission. The systems sustaining and translating the harmonious integration of impulses possess differing degrees of interaction with the physiology of the body. The most subtle interaction is probably that of gas concentrations outside the body with those inside the body. Atmospheric pressure plays a most important role in this exchange between gas and body fluids (ie, arterial and venous blood).

The second most basic interaction is the need for hydrostatic pressure to stimulate the functions inside the environment of the cell. The shear stress we find inside the blood vessel is perhaps the first expression of a mechanical interference between a "fluent mesoderm"[10] and its direct cellular environment.

Equally important are the needs of the cell population to create both an acid-base equilibrium and a hydro-electrical potential that is omnipresent. This is important not only at the cytoskeleton level, but also for the complete protein construction of the extracellular matrix of proteoglycans and collagen filaments.

We can conclude that the basic equilibrium of the body is guaranteed by equilibrium in atmospheric and hydrostatic pressures that interact on a cellular level with acid-base balance and hydro-electrical potential. For osteopaths, it is important to possess a comprehensive knowledge of these major systems of functioning, because if we succeed in understanding their interactions, we then have a good chance to re-establish homeostasis.

Should not an attentive osteopath avoid investigating the history of the patient's physical symptoms too exhaustively and instead focus on finding out which system/field is failing to integrate physiology? The renowned American osteopath Rollin Becker noted that symptoms and causes are not always related in a simple, straightforward manner.[11] The study of symptomatology and pathophysiology needs to stimulate the osteopath to attempt to *directly* feel and understand what is happening to the patient. We should accept a biomedical diagnosis only when we are unsuccessful in discovering the explanation for the alteration in physiology. Many symptoms should be interpreted as long-lasting attempts of the body to adapt to altered physiology, even if when they finally manifest themselves, they are isolated in time and in space from their source.

Is a simple hemorrhoid an expression of a local compression, a sign of local congestion, or an expression of portal hypertension? Is the portal hypertension dependent upon liver failure, or is it a precursor sign of an approaching cardiovascular incident?

Could it not be that portal hypertension and cardiovascular destabilization are both expressions of one and the same event—a subtle alteration of fluid exchange governed by a systemic deterioration?

Is it not so that abdominal hypertension interferes both locally and at a distance with the viscera and the cardiovascular physiology? Intrathoracic depression is determining for venous return to both the cranial sphere and the abdominal sphere. Restoring normal intrathoracic depression and abdominal pressures are keys for restoring health, by addressing subtle changes in specific tissue lesions impeding this vital exchange. The osteopath should think about which system is disorganized, rather than attempt to cope with an always-changing pattern of symptomatology.

When we succeed in changing the organization of the system/field, we have a good chance of making the symptoms disappear. If not, appropriate local and *technical techniques are needed.*

1.7 From symptom to compensation

It could be stated that coping with a symptom is a never-ending fight to find the origin of the attempt at compensation to accommodate the basic need for homeostasis. In other words, a system that risks destabilization in its physiology will try to establish a more complex interference with other systems capable of sustaining the threatened system. This is described well by Chauvet:

"If a structural unit is not capable of realizing its own elementary physiological function, then it needs to receive this function from an other structural unit possessing the qualities that can guarantee the survival of the threatened unit." [36]

We can suggest that compensatory phenomena and epiphenomena, as described in the osteopathic vocabulary, are possibly attempts to adapt physiology to a more normal state of function and survival. Could we not suppose, then, that by eliminating a compensation, we risk further destabilization of the system, should the normalization not be appropriate for the time schedule of the body? We need to better

---

[10] It was WG Sutherland who described the blood as a fluent mesoderm, perhaps indicating by this the mechanical function of blood on its environment, as confirmed in the work of PA Janmey

[11] Becker R. Life in Motion. Portland, OR: Stillness Press, 1997

understand the body's needs before trying to interfere with an altered physiology.

Two types of "brains" work out basic physiology:
- The first type has a well-established network of nerve)fibers that conduct impulses in a centripetal and centrifugal way between the brain and the periphery. This organization is a fast "highway," constructed for rapid adaptations and movement of information between the central nervous system (CNS) and the peripheral nervous system (PNS).
- The second type is a more disseminated brain, in that the cells of the immune system are dispersed throughout the body instead of being concentrated)in a localized place, such as the brain in the skull. This disseminated brain possesses a bony environment localized deeply in the bone marrow, where it is stimulated, and it is informed by cells from the periphery by means of colony-stimulating factors.

We can recognize a central organization and a peripheral organization. Different organs play well-defined roles in the coordination and integration of immune responses. Circulating B-cloned families and T-lymphocytes function as messengers between the periphery and the centralized germ layers, constantly informing the central organs (ie, the bone marrow and thymus). The most important peripheral organizations are linked to the gut and the peripheral lymph circuit, including the gut-associated lymphoid tissue (GALT), spleen, reticular-endothelial system (RES), and peripheral lymph nodes. As we can see, a major part of our adaptation is affected by these two functions. Basically, the CNS and PNS are the organizers of our fight-flight reaction pattern, and the lymphoid tissue organization is the organizer of our defense and integration pattern.

This concept attributes a cognitive function to the immune system instead of a purely defensive function. Evidence for this concept can be found in recent literature about psycho-neuro-immunology, including the works of Ader. [14] In analogous research, lymphocytic function is defined as the possibility of recognizing molecules that belong to the individual or that are alien to the individual on the basis of specific lymphocytic receptors. The former class of molecules are described as those of the self, and the latter class of molecules are those of the non-self, such as infectious agents. [39] In scientific literature, it is rare to find this hint of a more personalized description of biomolecular physiology. Perhaps this lack of content is a silent agreement to consider the immune system as a kind of specialized brain. This integrating part of our body system also has a fast adaptive organization, as almost the entire lymphocyte population changes every two days.

It is well known that almost all of the lymphocytes can activate a specific enzyme called recombinase, which is capable of changing the transcriptional modalities of its genome into a new adaptive reactive pattern upon variable external noxious stimuli.[12] The body is well-organized to establish rapid and effective adaptations that are integrated with body physiology. Once outside this adaptive capability, compensations must occur as attempts at reorganization.

Another consequence of this reorganization is that the biological system, which is searching for integration, adapts to the newly constructed reflex pathways with an altered reaction and integrative pattern. Many signals in the body that were previously interpreted as normal are now interpreted as harmful. In this way, physiology deviates from its normal pattern, displaying more and more auto-aggressive reaction patterns. Perhaps we should consider the autoimmune disorders as overcompensated patterns of adaptive physiology, which are not part of the genetic code of the individual.

This compensation, when summated with other compensations, can disable the normal integrative pattern of physiology and result in destabilization of all attempts of the organism to find homeostasis. Any shock at any level of integration can disorganize the adaptive possibility of the physiological systems of the body, forcing the body into altered behavior that integrates normally physiological stimuli into increasingly morbid behavior.

An interesting consideration is whether this type of compensation manifests itself only in tissue on a cellular level, where it can be fixed in altered reaction patterns or organizations (eg, as in fibrosis). Are the same changes also found in the behavior of the

---

[12] Gilbert SF. *Developmental Biology*. Sunderland, MA: Sinauer, 2003.

individual? Is human behavior a result of conditioned or adapted behavioral patterns—patterns that are considered normal because we cannot remember when they were inserted in our subconscious? Current concepts of psycho-neuro-immunology would consider these changes in cellular function and behavior to be part of the subconscious memory.

I would suggest that much of what we call behavior consists of complex adaptations to changing environments orientated by an invisible brain that is made up of the silent substratum of the informed tissue. In osteopathic practice, it is not unusual to see a person's life undergo a profound change following a simple normalization of the tissues. The question arises whether this change is an event that takes place in the patient's consciousness or whether it comes about due to altered reaction patterns in the tissues that are integrated into the patient's consciousness.

The holistic attitude of the European osteopath is geared toward viewing the human being as an individually functioning and reacting organism. Conditionals and questions are often used to underline this individuality. Tissue fixations, concentrations, and density[13] are able to direct the behavioral pattern of the individual in such a way that even the most unhealthy metabolic process is interpreted as normal on a physiological level. Perhaps this interpretation corresponds to the basic laws of osteopathy: absence of pain, support of economy, and equilibrium.

Apparently, the human body, like any biological system, possesses the ability to use stored energy for compensation purposes, if necessary. The body also has the intrinsic ability to convert its accumulated potential energy into a kinetic energy, a process accompanied intimately by heat production, which we can call a state of increased entropy. We can suppose that memory is not as conscious as we usually think of it. Apart from the important role the brain plays in actualizing memory and compensation patterns, the immune system seems at least as important to

body consciousness as the rapid adaptations of the brain.

Each tissue is built upon a structure that retains in its configuration adaptive and integrated patterns belonging to different space/time units. These units are fixed in biochemical, biomechanical, and bioelectrical patterns appropriate to particulare tissues, helping the structure to expose specific adaptive and integrative cues.

The brain is built upon tissue histories developed throughout an individual's lifetime, in such a way that it knows all of the contents and facts that impact tissue and express themselves as feelings/sensations.[14] Brain memory is, in a certain sense, an extremely complex collection of tissue/cell information that is integrated in increasingly intricate forms of memory combinations and patterning.

1.8 From molecular organization to body orientation

When we examine a patient, we try to interpret function from the form or movement we perceive with our hands. Do we have to accept that the patient can be defined by what his or her form is displaying; a patchwork of physiological events and symptoms? Is man only form or subtle movements perceived by specialized therapists? Are form and movement nothing more than an expression of subtler proceedings happening at the molecular level?

Molecular biology can teach us much about how form and movement express deeper layers of the dynamic organization of the body, invisible to the naked eye. Only logic and observation can teach us that every living being is preferentially orientated in space, exhibiting a preponderant pattern of movements organized and summated by the micromovements of cells and molecules.

Hegstrom and Kondpudi [40] describe how molecules can be chiral, displaying D-enantiomeres and

---

13 J Upledger calls it "energetic cysts." See *Craniosacral Therapy.* Seattle, WA: Eastland Press, 1983.

14 Damasio A. *L'autre moi-même.* Paris, France: Odile Jacob, 2010.

L-enantiomeres—L and D standing for left (levo) and right (dexter). Enantiomeric forms are found in many organic and inorganic substances. They are essentially in all molecules crucial for the development of life-specific proteins. Among the several hundred amino acids that exist, only 20 amino acids—specifically L-amino acids—make up all proteins. The main function of the proteins called enzymes is to catalyze biomolecular reactions, including the synthesis of other proteins. The catalytic ability of enzymes depends on their three-dimensional structure, which, in turn, depends on their L-amino sequence.

Because of the combinations of its key molecules, human chemistry is highly sensitive to enantiomeric differences, such as the molecular enantiomeric orientation of certain medications (eg, thalidomide) and possibly of certain food compounds. DNA-RNA nucleic acids also possess a preferential chirality determined by the presence of D-sugars exhibiting a right-handed helix. Is it not amazing that the outer environment of the cell (ie, the membrane) as well as the cytoplasm organelles and extracellular matrix are all structured by left-orientated helices, while the nucleus is organized by a right-handed helix?

It is probable that the equilibrium of a cell is determined by a balance between right- and left-handed helices—that is, a specific balance between right- and left-orientating molecular organizations. If we remember that the complete embryological event is a continuing exchange of nuclear (ie, genetic) information and cellular environmental information, then it is not so astonishing that this event is reflected and reused at every biomolecular and atomic level that supports the continued transformation of different body fields during adult life.

The macro form of the body's organization displays the memory of this subtle equilibrium. As the authors describe, human beings are structurally chiral, with the heart to the left of center and the liver to the right. The liver, involved in such major metabolic activities as glycogenolysis and neoglycogenesis, is particularly dependent upon the quality of the introduced sugars, especially the D-sugars. The heart, as a muscle, metabolizes catabolic products, such as lactic acid. In embryology, the heart fulfills the active and rhythmic propelling of the metabolic activity of the liver toward the developing brain (hepatization-cardialization-cerebralization). Would it be wrong to consider the liver as the inner information of the developing body and the heart as a response upon outer metabolic needs, provoking rhythm and orientation, as proposed by Blechschmidt and Gasser? [19]

As long as the right chiral orientation of the liver (D-sugars) and the left chiral function of the heart (enzymatic activity, systolic propulsion) are equilibrated, the body is able to express homeostasis.

Even the predominant right-handedness of humans seems to depend upon the subtle and deep-layered effect of molecular and atomic organization.[15] Subtle enzymatic processing may temporarily disturb any equilibrium, ranging from biomolecular to biomechanical functions.

It is unknown if simple compressive or stretching techniques on an organ or on the whole body could influence the subtle spiral orientation of biomolecular and biomechanical functions. However, studying the simplest biodynamical movements of tissue and viscera during the embryological and fetal developmental phases allows for greater understanding of the importance of these dynamics for the spatial orientation of the developing individual. Even the birth process is a continuation of the earlier established spiral rotations. The whole body, from skull to pelvis, is impregnated by the first rotation it underwent during the passage through the birth canal.

We could suggest that all vital events—ranging from molecular to enzymatic to mechanical—are fully impregnated by these spiral orientations, partly by their geometrical proportions and partly by their mechanics.

1.9 The spiral organization of the body and its implications on function and disease

The body, in its dimensionality, has been described as having different axes—longitudinal, transversal, and anterior-posterior—which intersect in every component of the body. Most of the time, these axes

---

[15] The dominance of the right hand over the left hand is universal, independent of race or culture. [39]

have been used solely as biomechanical tools or as orientations for the anatomical descriptive nomenclature. In fact, they serve only to direct descriptive essays of the body at rest or in motion.

In more advanced biomechanical research, it has become clear that the so-called axes function more like fluctuating, hyperbolic lines—that is, a succession, in time and space, of changing points that construct a certain line of articular, biomechanical evolution of a specific joint, organ, or flux.

We can state that axes are, for the greatest part, functional representations instead of functional constancy. This does not correspond with the observation that a biological system preferentially uses chaos (symmetry in the quantum concept) to express the full functioning of its components, with entropy being a physical indicator of progress and direction of the exchange with the environment. Its evolution is accompanied by thermodynamic changes that will be fully or partially recuperated.[16]

The anatomical and biochemical organization of the biological environment of the body clearly illustrates that there exists a more substantial and fundamental organization, integrating function in a subtle manner at all levels of physical interaction, from the most basic biomechanical level to the most profound biochemical level. In other words, what happens at a biochemical level profoundly interferes with preferential organizations of biomechanical functions and vice versa.

Schmitt W.H. [41] mentioned the close relationship that exists between torque patterns of the body and a vast array of immune and biochemical functions that influence health or illness. In his studies on electron poising curves, he described two patterns of body functioning coinciding with different responses upon enzymatic and hormonal levels. The clockwise rotating pattern (CW) and the counterclockwise rotating pattern (CCW) each express a predisposition for certain types of physiological responses and illness patterns. CCW, or right foot torque patterns, seem to suppress the immune system, while the CW, or left foot torque, enhances immune responses. For example, CCW seems to predispose the individual to cancer and HIV

sensibility, and CW predisposes the individual to autoimmune disorders and allergy.

Norepinephrine activates the second messenger system inside the cell (ie, c-AMP[17]) and induces suppression of the immune system. [42] Serotonin activates c-GMP and enhances the immune system. The endocrine system is governed by the same patterns, so that the CCW rotation decreases pineal gland function and increases pituitary function. In addition, thyroid and steroid functioning are both increased. In the CW rotation, there is an increased pineal function with a dampening of the steroid and thyroid function.

By influencing these patterns through specific manipulative techniques, the osteopath may be able to change, in a more or less definite way, the illness predisposition of the patient. In other words, the biochemistry of the body, with its predisposing orientation to illness, could be influenced by specific mechanical corrective measures. The osteopathic techniques presented by Masters [1] in the model of Gordon Zinc are all focused upon unwinding the different diaphragms of the body. Results of those techniques may be the most valuable indicators that the rotational pattern of a given diaphragm is an important determinant in both physiological and pathological patterns.[18]

The domed structures of the body are witnesses of the structural and functional adaptation of body and function to three-dimensionality. Isn't it true that ocular movements or auditory-dependent head positions determine a specific pattern of head and neck torque, elicited by oculo-cephalo-gyric or vestibulogyric reflexes? And isn't it also true that head position,

---

[16] It is stated that functional organization begins at the borderline of chaos.

[17] The intracellular second messenger system, for example, seems to play a major role in the generation of asthmatic attacks. Activation of phospholipase C or adenylate cyclase create, respectively, an increase in intracellular calcium or an increase in c-AMP, enhancing or diminishing spasm of the bronchial muscles. Could it be possible that the osteopath, by altering the diaphragmatic orientations (left or right torque), influences this liberation of mediators—and sustains or inhibits the allergenic or spastic reactions of the respiratory tissue?

[18] Zinc defined various possible patterns of adaptation of the body to gravity—including a common compensated pattern, an uncommon compensated pattern, an uncompensated pattern, and a rare, free pattern.

whether or not influenced by these reflexes, predisposes the body to biomechanical adaptations at all levels?

Consider that the entire body is squeezed in a spiral way by uterus contractions during the process of birth, with the skull being the first structure to undergo a rotational pattern during this process. As a result, there probably is a certain predisposition for illness that is inserted into the physical program of the individual, exclusively by the way the body was expelled when it was born.

Apparently, illness is not only a matter of genetic predisposition or environmental influences, but also an expression of spatially and mechanically integrated body patterns. He who is able to interfere with the mechanical pattern may also be able to interfere with the illness predisposition of the genome.[19, 20] In other words, the osteopath is not really healing the body, but balancing the body toward a better level of adaptation to disturbing factors.

Another interesting question arises: how are these adaptive torque patterns to gravity counterbalanced by more intrinsic body organizations? The major external perceivable torque should be equilibrated by structures other than only the myofascial organization serving the biomechanical integrity. Indeed, the internal fascial structure pattern is conceived in such a way that it displays a subtle organization of interfering three-dimensional rotation patterns of organs, which interact by fascial articulations, as mentioned in the work of Barral. [43, 44]

Great parts of these fascial articulations are remnants, or memories, of embryological structuring.[21] This means that a great deal of the body's functioning is based upon, or is an adapted rehearsal of, these construction patterns. As Crutchfield et al [45] state, structure is not only characterizing an actual state of function in space, but it is also the expression of the dynamics of changing states in time.

Mutations in the genetic material could be conceived of as progressive adaptations to subtle long-lasting external information that, at any given moment, is able to switch to an adapted pattern of functioning. This is another reason to believe that what we call treatment could be a false belief that we reinstall the original state of health. Treatment probably contributes to a new pattern of adaptation by adding new information to the tissue. Treatment is similar to the illness-inducing pattern—every time a stimulus is added to the structure, the structure is obliged to transform and integrate the stimulus, whether it is a manipulation or an incubation of a germ.

From this point of view, treatment informs more than it treats a dysfunctional state of the body. It permits the body to accumulate potential energy and to convert it in contribution to adaptation patterns inherent to the disabled area. We do not treat, we add—we inform the body about the ever-existing possibility of adaptation that is hidden in the tissue.

The question may arise why methods of informing, or of curing, people are necessary? The answer is simple, in that an added energy can be integrated only into an already existing pattern of structuring. At brain level, it is called the basic state of the receptive field (➤ Fig. 1.3). The tissue level is organized by, and interacting through, the electrical field in which biochemical cybernetic exchange is taking

---

[19] On the other hand, one should not deny the importance of genetically determined abnormalities in growth, form, or function of the cortex as factors organizing the birth process in time and space. Swaab D, in his book *Wij zijn ons brein* (*We are our brain*), mentions that brain deficiencies installed at the embryonic period play an important role in the way the birth process and later functional abnormalities will be expressed. (Swaab D. *Wij zijn ons brein*. Netherlands: Atlas-Contact, 2010)

[20] Freeman B talks about "windows of opportunity" (as do other embryological articles) and developmental phases that facilitate tissue differentiation and specification during embryological development, orientating the ability of the body for adaptation during postnatal life. (Freeman B. *Sutherland Cranial College Magazine*, issue 32, 2010.)

[21] About the cellular development during embryology, Barral states the following:

"*Ces cellules ont un ordre bien défini dans l'espace et le temps. Il existe un coordinateur qui les fera s'aligner et se développer en toute harmonie. La cellule est une mémoire.*"

About fascial movement he states, "*Ces mouvements sont inscrits dans les fibres viscérales, la théorie embryologique consiste à dire que le tissu viscéral a gardé cette mémoire et que les mouvements viscéraux s'effectuent de part et d'autre d'une position embryonnaire et un retour à la position d'origine, avec une contractilité qui pourrait être analogue à celle du tissu nodal du coeur.*"

place. The whole is converted in an electromagnetic potency that sustains structure and rhythm, creating the phenomenon of resonance between different structures, organs, and possibly individuals.

This physiology takes place inside pre-existing patterns of structural organization that display direction, depth, and rhythm, enabling the therapist to discover the so-called patterns of dysfunction.

At the level of biochemical exchange, the same is true, with a substantial part of the reaction pattern taking place in one specialized tissue that always displays the same properties of adaptation—the mesenchyme. It is from out of this tissue that the fibroblast cells originate. These cells continue to function as totipotential adapters to continuously changing needs of function and structure. They are the remnants of this embryological important tissue that interfered with all integration changes of newly obtained function and emplacement of organs and body systems.

The cytokine system (eg, interleukins, TNFα, TNFβ) is integrated in almost every cell that sustains a certain function of messaging, including leukocytes, macrophages, lymphocytes, monocytes, and fibroblasts. This system is perhaps the most messenger active of all systems, both in physiological processes and pathological processes.

The spiral patterns that we find among the torque patterns of the whole body, turning to the left or to the right, are possibly the most subtle and elaborated constructions of three-dimensionality in life. They permit the human body to integrate intelligence, affection, emotion, and physical components in one and the same pattern of organization integrated at the tissue level. This means that the same electromagnetic and biochemical field can simultaneously serve to sustain intelligence and biomechanical functioning—or, by the principle of resonance, it can affect an organ in its rhythm by simple emotional disturbance.

The same is also true for an externally added force, such as a therapeutic maneuver. The force certainly follows one of the already inserted paths in the structure, but it can do so in a recurrent way or in a progressive way. Both the recurrent and the progressive ways are capable of initiating different types of reactions by the same pattern of resonance. A simple manipulation of an organ can induce physiological patterns as it also elicits emotional patterns. Most osteopaths have made this observation at least once.

To treat the body could mean that we enable the body to adapt better to changing circumstances, once by liberating an old, fixed memory and once by freeing it from a hidden disturbance in its biochemical, biomechanical, or electromagnetic field. The longer these nameless fixations reside in the body, the more they get a chance to be fixed in a cognitive pattern. In the short term, all disturbances are in a certain way traumatic, because they disturb the current pattern of adaptation at the different levels of physical integration. Trauma could be reduced to the level of physical organization of the structure that organizes fields of interaction between different systems of functioning. It is reducible to biochemical or electromagnetic field disturbances, which interfere with every level of structural and hierarchical organization, ranging from the cellular-extracellular matrix interference to the highest and most complex psycho-emotional patterns of expression.

It is Heine [46] in his book on biological medicine, who mentions the possibility of superposition of different webs of organization in the biological field— and who also indicates the existence of cybernetic cycles of interaction between distinct disturbing fields (focal patterns). By means of these organizations, one field of dysfunction can become the organizer of a different field that expresses its pathology independently from the earlier existing symptoms of the inductive field.[22] Illness could be a fractal of a preexisting predisposition of a certain type of reactivity of tissue, organ, or cell on an added stimulus. This property is defined as *pre-tension* (Vorspannung).

It is the pre-tension that predisposes the individual to a certain type of illness, because this tension is typical for a type of tissue that has already become the target for information varying from genetic programming to environmental aggression. At each level, the organs/cells react with the same array of cybernetic messaging by autocrine, paracrine, juxtacrine, endocrine or intracrine transmission. In most cases, cell-to-cell interactions are mediated by cytokines, which, together with the fundamental

---

22 Die Berücksichtigung kybernetischer Zusammenhänge zwingt, den Boden monokausalen Denkens zu verlassen. In der Medizin wird daher der Weg der Wissenschaftlichkeit verlassen, wenn versucht wird, eindimensionale Kausalketten auf vernetzte Systeme anzuwenden.

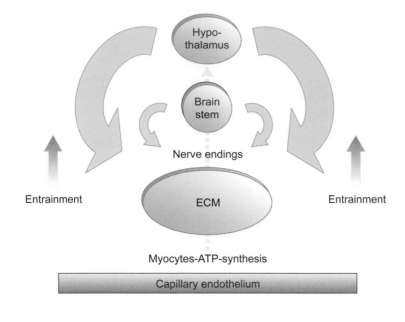

Fig. 1.3 Regulation of autonomous control by deep brain centers upon extracellular matrix (ECM)

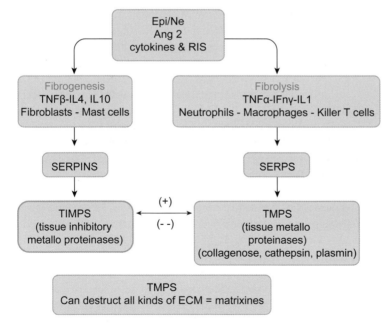

Fig. 1.4 Tissue inflammatory processes are governed by tissue enzymes in interferences with cytokines and local endocrine substance concentrations.

substance (extracellular matrix), contain the space-time memory of the tissue. They are the mediators between fibroblasts, lymph cells, and the mesenchyme. Even proteoglycans possess cytokine activity in certain areas of their protein construction. [46]

We could say that the fibroblast has a more specialized embryological memory of transformed mes-

enchyme tissue than is incorporated in distinct organ functions. It is, at the same time, the only structure that offers an almost immediate answer upon changing cellular and tissue environments, by producing new glycosaminoglycans (GAG's) and proteoglycans (PG's). In this way, the mesenchyme, as part of the extracellular matrix, is a continuous

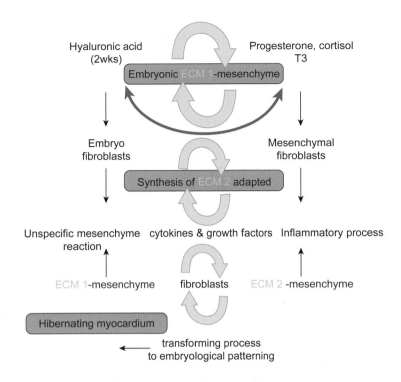

Fig. 1.5 Inflammatory processes can induce a reiteration of ontogenetic differentiation of tissue, such as the "hibernating of myocardium."

expression of chemomechanical modeling induced by internal and external environmental impulses.

Reckoning with what Heine mentioned, it could be possible that the immediate tissue adaptation is in accord with previously made adaptations, building in this way a time-space relationship in the body memory that exceeds the simple linear cause-symptom relationship of pathology. It is, for example, now clear that fibroblasts and the depending mesenchyme can activate an embryological pattern if necessary. Metalloproteinases and their inhibitors could play a decisive role in switching from one type of program to another, embryological program, depending upon the kinds of cytokines that are segregated (➤ Fig. 1.4, ➤ Fig. 1.5).

1.10 The life of cells: a cyclic behavior

Osteopathy considers "vital force" as the origin of all physiological events of the body, generating no-

tions of function, motion, strength and rhythm. A major part of diagnostics in osteopathy is based upon the evaluation and quantification of motion and rhythm. Motion could be interpreted as mechanical mobility, motility (involuntary mobility), or vital motility (motion of cells and tissue not quantifiable until now, but suggesting a certain degree of vitality).

Sutherland defined these rather physical parameters of vitality as motion, amplitude, and rhythm, and he referred to the "Tide" as the big motor of life force and expression of the "Breath of Life." It is amazing that an osteopath can refer to such a wide range of diagnostic tools and still agree with colleagues about the patient's diagnosis. These three parameters can all be sensed by manual palpation without reference to mechanical tools to quantify, resulting in agreement about diagnosis or possible ways to treat.

The question arises if motion is generated by rhythm, or if rhythm is generated by motion. Is the primary respiratory mechanism (PRM) defined by Sutherland an expression of rhythm or of motion? Is the palpating hand perceiving motion, rhythm, or vibration.?[23]

- Rhythm could be considered an expression of co-herency of different physiological phases at work during a specific body event. For example, fleeing from a charging tiger could express a completely different coherency in the brain field than reading a romantic story.

- Motion could be considered the resultant of different physical and biochemical patterns at work during a specific program of expression or integration of information.

Motion and rhythm seem to be ideal expressions of an inherent space-time relationship hidden within the secrets of living tissue. They permit quantifiable evaluations as well as more subjective evaluations of changes in such parameters as depth, direction, amplitude, and force of expression. Research conducted upon the tool of evaluation, namely the hand, evokes similar ambiguity. The hand is capable of perceiving micromovements at the borderline of vibration information[24]

We could ask if the brain interprets motional information rather than vibration information, or if it integrates both at the same time to establish a right image of perception and representation? Quantification may refer to the two parameters when interpreted separately, and qualification (as a subjective parameter) may refer to a mixture of these two ways of signaling. When we conceive of motion and rhythm at a cellular level, we could note that cells are capable of vibrating in a dynamic manner with complex harmonics, which can now be measured and analyzed in a quantitative manner by Fourier analysis. [47]

DNA breathing is well established, and nucleotides in DNA sequences have been shown to oscillate according to their base pair compositions, as mentioned by Pienta et al. [30] Those authors further mention that proteins vibrate in the range of 1012 to 1015 times per second. The physiological significance of these oscillations is that, for example, the vibrations of the myoglobin molecule allow for the transport of oxygen in and out of the protein. It is also believed that protein structural vibrations are important components of enzyme active sites. Ions oscillating between intracellular or intercellular compartments have been demonstrated in several systems. In Purkinje cells, the oscillations of calcium ions across the cell membrane causes the rhythm of the heartbeat. [48, 49]

Biological oscillations also occur during other cellular processes. For example, the mechanisms involved in the control of the periodicity of the mitotic cycle have been partially elucidated.[25] Elements within the nucleus and cytoplasm appear to be coupled in a coordinated manner between a nuclear cycle and a cytoplasmatic cycle. Cell mitosis is activated by a nuclear maturation promoting factor (or mitosis promoting factor) (MPF),[26] which is controlled by cellular-plasmatic oscillations. Those oscillations are capable of interrupting MPF activity in a cyclic manner and organizing the oscillations of cells.[27] Cyclin, a cytoplasmatic protein, could be the activator of the MPF. This protein displays cyclic phases of plasmatic concentration and plasmatic dilution. [50]

These cell vibrations and intracellular oscillations are essential for the biochemical equilibrium of the cell and its environment. They are also essential for determining carcinogenesis and other disturbances of organized cell apoptosis. [30, 51]

The entire system of cell oscillation and rhythm seems to be dependent upon physical factors capable of transmitting chemomechanical signals from the cell to its extracellular matrix and vice versa. We have previously described the mechanism of this signaling under the heading of tensegrity.

One can imagine the impact of these "thinking fingers" on all levels of the functioning of cells and extracellular matrix (ECM), including pure molecular signaling, over chemical coding, genetic coding, and mechanical transferring. A most important fact for the osteopath is that a mechanical approach toward the body interferes with almost all of the subtle signaling mechanisms of the cell and its environment.

---

[23] Sutherland talked about "feeling, thinking, knowing fingers." Sutherland WG. *Contributions of Thought: The Collected Writings of Willian Garner Sutherland*. Fort Worth, TX: Sutherland Cranial Teaching Foundation, 1998.
[24] See footnot 23.

[25] Oscillations in MPF and its subcomponents of cyclin and and cdc-2 kinase play a critical role in the timing of events within the mitotic cycle.
[26] MPF is also the activating substance during cell meiosis.
[27] The interphase during c.ell divisions could be conceived of as an expression of this cyclic behavior of the cell.

Two dynamics—the patient and the therapist—probably interfere with each other, displaying aspects of their particularity under different mechanical parameters, such as strength, tension, warmth, rhythm, and vibratory impulses.

If we consider cell vitality, we can note that vibration in the cell organizes cyclic patterns of functioning, in which motion is included. The hand possesses different receptors, which can perceive these evolutions in a kinesthetic and proprioceptive manner. A mixture of deforming forces arising from both the surface of the skin (external deformation) and changes in tissue pressure within the dermis (internal deformation) are interpreted as mechanical inputs orientating mechano-perception.

Most of the corpuscles are specialized in perception of motion, but one kind is specialized in the perception of variations of frequencies. Meissner's corpuscles are associated with quickly adapting mechanoreceptor fibers and are velocity active. Slowly adapting fibers I are associated with Merkel cells, and slowly adapting fibers II are related to Ruffini's end organs. Pacinian fibers respond to high frequency (200-300 Hz) vibratory stimuli, complementing the 20-40 Hz response range of the quickly adapting fibers.

One can remark that the perception of frequencies induces the notion of mechanical displacement. Recent research confirms the possibility of the multifunctional potential of Merkel cells[28] for displaying a role in electromagnetic reception, fingerprint formation, epigenetic inheritance, and hair form. These data suggest that perceptual tools developed by the body during its functional exchange with its immediate environment could guide tactile perception. Vibratory perception and electromagnetic perception could have been two exquisite properties of the perceptual field of the body in preventing danger by aggressors or heat (burning).

This information constitutes a perceptual field that informs the brain about other qualities of interference in addition to the usual tactile and proprioceptive cues. The subconscious perception of these interferences may be linked to the creation of coherency phases in the body (the brain) of the therapist, enabling him or her to interpret some invisible clinical cues as valuable additions for making up the diagnostic uptake of the patient's condition. I will try to explain this further in chapter 9 by focusing on the use of the mental image in the osteopathic approach to the patient.

A fusion between the rhythms of the patient and the perceptor creates the possibility of interpreting the physiology of the patient. For example, Norton [52] proposes a "tissue pressure model" to explain the perceived notion of cranial rhythmic impulse (CRI) throughout the body. The sensation described as CRI is related to activation of slowly adapting cutaneous mechanoreceptors by tissue pressures of both the examiner and the patient. The sources of change in these tissue pressures are the combined respiratory and cardiovascular rhythms of both examiner and patient. This CRI is expressed throughout the body by all tissues that integrate changes in arterial pressure (dependent upon the pumping action of the heart) and changes in venous pressure (generated by intrathoracic pressure fluctuations).[29]

Norton further indicates that when sensory input related to the temperature, texture, movements, and pressures within the tissues is obtained through palpation and combined with information from other sensory modalities, a complex picture of the patient's physiological state emerges: "*Much of the sensory input and integration takes place below the level of consciousness. Part of the difficulty in discussing*

---

28 Merkel cells are located in glabrous and hairy skin and in some mucosa. They are characterized by dense core secretory granules and cytoskeletal elements. They are attached to neighboring keratinocytes by desmo.somes, and they contain melanosomes, similar to keratinocytes. These melanosomes seem to be involved in mammalion magnetoreception. The melanosome can be considered as a biological magnetite that is connected by cytoskeletal filaments to mechanically gated ion channels embedded in the Merkel cell membrane. Movement of the melanosome with a changing electromagnetic field may open ion channels, producing a receptor potential that can be transmitted to the brain via sensory neurons.
Irmak MK. Multifunctional Merkel cell(s): their roles in electromagnetic reception, finger-print formation, Reiki, epigenetic inheritance and hair form. Med Hypotheses. 2010;75:162-168.

---

29 Fryman VM states the following: "It may be contended with some force of argument that the apparent sensation of a slow cranial rhythm represents only a 'beat' frequency between, say, the two pulse cycles." A study of the rhythmic motions of the living cranium. *J Am Osteopath Assoc.* 1971;70:928-945.

*palpatory results may be due to the nonverbal charac-
ter of the palpatory diagnostic process."*

In a different sense, we could state that what is
called palpation by the examiner is indirectly a source of information for the patient's tissues. Palpation,
defined in the sense of synchronization of two
rhythms, could have the effect of holographic
transcription of the physiologic state of the patient
to the therapist, and vice versa. The more the therapist is able to accept different rhythms at his own
tissue level, the more information he can obtain
from the patient's tissues. In addition, such properties as tear, pull, stretch, vibration, heat, and cold,
which are transmitted involuntarily by the palpating
hand, could be codetermining factors for the quality
of the therapeutic maneuver.

REFERENCES

[1] Masters P. Theoretical and practical implications of the
respiratory and circulatory model of Gordon Zinc in osteopathy. Presented at a conference; 1998; Namur,
Beligium.

[2] Blechschmidt E. Wie Beginnt das Menschliche Leben.
Stein am Rein, Germany: Christiana-Verlag, 1989.

[3] Morgon RA, Dubbins PA. Pancreatic and renal mobility. Clin Radiol. 1992;45(2):88–91.

[4] Blomström-Lundqvist C, et al. Ventricular dimensions
and wall motion assessed by echocardiography in patients with arrhytmogenic right ventricular dysplasia.
Eur Heart J. 1998;9(12):1291–1302.

[5] Wallis TW, et al. Mechanical heart-lung interaction
with positive end-expiratory pressure. J Appl Physiol
Respir Environ Exerc Physiol. 1983;54(4):1039–1047.

[6] Aubert AE, et al. Contactless detection of heart movements with a laser. Acta Cardiol. 1988;43(3):263–267.

[7] Bryan PJ, et al. Respiratory movement of the pancreas:
an ultrasonic study. J Ultrasound Med. 1984;3(7):317–
320.

[8] Prandota J, Ostrowska-Skora J. Normal limits for renal
mobility in children. Int J Pediatr Nephrol.
1984;5(3):171–174.

[9] Suramo I, et al. Cranio-caudal movements of the liver,
pancreas and kidneys in respiration. Acta Radiol Di-
agn. 1984;25(2):129–131.

[10] Korin HW, et al. Respiratory kinematics of the upper
abdominal organs: a quantitative study. Magn Reson
Med. 1992;23(1):172–178.

[11] Moerland MA, et al. The influence of respiration induced motion of the kidneys on the accuracy of radiothe-
rapy treatment planning, a magnetic resonance imaging study. Radiother Oncol. 1994;30(2):150–154.

[12] Schwartz LH et al. Kidney mobility during respiration.
Radiother Oncol. 1994;32(1):84–86.

[13] Prandota J, Sidor D. Urographic percentile charts for
vertical kidney mobility in childhood. Intl Urol Nephrol.
1996;28(1):1996.

[14] Davies SC, et al. Ultrasound quantitation of respiratory
organ motion in the upper abdomen. Br J Radiol.
1994;67(803):1096–1102.

[15] Arnerlov C, et al. Renal mobility in clinical patient material submitted for urography. Scand J Urol Nephrol.
1998;32(3):181–185.

[16] Rakusin A, et al. Intraperitoneal renal transplant mobility: the transposed transplant. Clin Nucl Med.
1999;24(7):530–531.

[17] Aoki C, Siekevitz P. Plasticity in brain development. Sci
Am. 1988;259(6):56–64.

[18] Pischinger A. Das Schicksal der Leukozyten. Z Mikrosk
Anat Forsch. 1957;63(2):169–192.

[19] Blechschmidt E, Gasser RF. Biokinetics and Biodyna-
mics of Human Differentiation. Springfield, IL: Charles
Thomas Publishing, 1978.

[20] Ghassemzadeh-Haddadi N. Grundlagen für eine "komplementäre" Akupunktur. Dtsch Zschr Akup.
1987;5:100–108.

[21] Carlson BM. Human Embryology and Developmental
Biology. St Louis, MO: Mosby-Year Book, 1994.

[22] Pischinger A. Das System der Grundregulation. Heidelberg, Germany: Haug Verlag, 1985.

[23] Lamers HJ. Het grondsysteem volgens Pischinger. Congres on Neuraltherapie; 1985; Utrecht, Netherlands.

[24] Ader R, ed. Psychoneuroimmunology. New York City,
NY: Elsevier Academic Press, 1981.

[25] Huneke F. Das Sekundenphänomen. Heidelberg, Germany: Haug Verlag, 1975.

[26] Janmey PA. The cytoskeleton and cell signaling: component localization and mechanical coupling. Physiol
Rev. 1998;78(3):763–782.

[27] Ingber DE, et al. Cellular tensegrity: exploring how
mechanical changes in the cytoskeleton regulate cell
growth, migration, and tissue pattern during morphogenesis. Int Rev Cytol. 1994;150:173–224.

[28] Ingber DE. Cellular tensegrity: defining new rules of
biological design that govern the cytoskeleton. J Cell
Sci. 1993;104(Pt 3):613–627.

[29] Stamenovic D, et al. A microstructural approach to cytoskeletal mechanics based on tensegrity. J Theor Biol.
1996;181(2):125–136.

[30] Pienta KJ, Coffey DS. Cellular harmonic information
transfer through a tissue tensegrity-matrix system.
Med Hypotheses. 1991;34(1):88–95.

[31] Gumbiner BM. Cell adhesion: the molecular basis of
tissue architecture and morphogenesis. Cell.
1996;84(3):345–357.

[32] Wang N, et al. Mechanotransduction across the cell
surface and through the cytoskeleton. Science.
1993;260(5111):1124–1127.

[33] Ingber DE. Tensegrity: the architectural basis of cellular mechantransduction. Ann Rev Physiol.
1997;59:575–599.

[34] Ingber DE. Integrins as mechanochemical transducers. Curr Opin Cell Biol. 1991;3(5):841–848.

[35] Guan JL, Chen HC. Signal transduction in cell-matrix interactions. Int Rev Cytol. 1996;168:81–121.

[36] Chauvet G. La vie dans la matière. Paris, France: Flammarion, 1995.

[37] Ghassemzadeh-Haddadi N. Spezielle neuroembryonale Grundlagen für die komplementäre Akupunktur. Dtsch Zchr Akup. 1990;33:124–128.

[38] Von Vareka J, Richter E. Enzymatischer Schutz im Organismus als integrierter Bestandteil des Immunsystems. Natur Heilpraxis. 1992;4:411–418.

[39] Ameisen J-C. Le suicide des cellules. Pour la Science. 1996;Juin 96:52,53.

[40] Hegstrom RA, Kondepudi DK. The handedness of the universe. Sci Am. 1990;262(1):98–105.

[41] Schmitt WH. The effects of gait and torque on enhancing and suppressing immune system function. In: Centering the Spine. Shawnee Mission, KS: International College of Applied Kinesiology, 1987:259–279, 353–379.

[42] Ganong WF. Inositol trisphophate and cyclic AMP as second messengers. In: Ganong's Review of Medical Physiology. Appleton & Lange, 1995:37–39.

[43] Barral JP, Mercier P. Manipulations viscérales. Tôme 1. Paris, France: Maloine, 1983.

[44] Barral JP. Manipulations viscérales II. Paris, France: Maloine, 1987.

[45] Crutchfield JP, et al. Chaos. Heidelberg, Germany: Spektrum der Wissenschaft, 1987:78–90.

[46] Heine H. Lehrbuch der biologischen Medizin. Stuttgart, Germany: Hippokrates Auflage, 1997:13–45.

[47] Partin AW, et al. Early cell motility changes associated with an increase in metastatic ability in rat prostatic cancer cells transfected with the v-Harvey-ras oncogene. Cancer Res. 1998:48(21):6050.

[48] Nieman CJ, Eisner DA. Effects of caffeine, tetracaine, and ryanodine on calcium-dependent oscillations in sheep cardiac Purkinje fibers. J Gen Physiol. 1985;86(6):877–879.

[49] Lakatta EG. Functional implications of spontaneous sarcoplasmic reticulum Ca2+ release in the heart. Cardiovasc Res. 1992;26(3):193–214.

[50] Murray AW, Kirschner MW. Wie Proteine den Zellzyklus steuern. Heidelberg, Germany: Spektrum der Wissenschaft, 1991:126–131.

[51] Ameisen J-C. Le suicide des cellules. Pour la Science. 1996;Juin 96:54–59.

[52] Norton JM. A tissue pressure model for palpatory perception of the cranial rhythmic impulse. J Am Osteopath Assoc. 1991;91(10):975–977,980.

2

Neural crest cells and migrating mesothelial cells: organizers of structure, form, and function

2.1 Preliminary remarks

A considerable part of this review on the interactions of neural crest and epithelio-mesenchymal interaction is based upon two main studies. The work of B.M. Carlson and that of E. Blechschmidt and R.F. Gasser provided the basic materials to structure this chapter. Their references are mentioned later in this article. Additional important information was found in the work of N. Le Dourain, who conducted much of her scientific research in tracing the migratory pathways of neural crest cells (NCC's) in chick and quail chimeras.

Biodynamic and biokinetic developmental features expressed during cell and tissue differentiation are completely analogous and synchronic with the biomolecular differentiation that guides epithelio-mesenchymal and ectomesenchymal exchanges during embryonic development. The synchronous progression between molecular exchange patterns and the biodynamic and biokinetic modeling of structure and organs underlines the importance of the mechanical way of interfering with tissue. Mechanics not only interfere with the biomechanical aspects of life (ie, mobility, joint play, motion, and motility), but they are synchronous manifestations of biophysical and biochemical processes. They may interfere with each other in a bidirectional manner and are necessarily linked.

These synchronous manifestations of biophysical and biochemical processes can be referred to in osteopathic terminology as the "drug store" that A.T. Still related intimately to the mechanics of the body. Their synergism is sustained by the qualifying force of the "bio-energy" mentioned by R.E. Becker. The "great supervisor" is represented by "The Tide" that integrates rhythm, force, and balanced exchange.

One may ask about the usefulness of these biochemical and biophysical cues in the manual approach

to the body as practiced in osteopathy. Osteopaths have to find the link between the molecular, submolecular, and macroscopic events of motility and mobility. That's the reason one must study embryology, morphology, and their dynamics—to fully understand the secrets of inductive and differentiation processes at the very beginning of tissue differentiation.

The best link I have found between embryology and mechanics is probably represented by the work of L.V. Beloussov.[1]

Beloussov referred to each morphological differentiation of tissue during embryogenesis as an expression of "protest" against its mechanical deformation. This could mean that each tissue state prefers to stay in its original constellation—something that is verifiable when one studies the stress/strain curves of tissue during deformation. One could almost conclude that each important moment of tissue deformation is experienced as a kind of elastic recoil toward its original state of differentiation.

Each state can be considered as a physical and biochemical "momentum" that could serve as memory, referential to later occurring deformations and transformations. This protest could be considered as a primary memory.

What osteopaths call "shifting points of balance" may refer to the sensations of different shifts at multiple tissue levels that repeat, in a synchronous way, passages of important transformation of their biochemical and biophysical states, which refer to the history of their integrated and evolutionary functions. The tissue contains many such organizers that determine parts of its evolutionary development. Lymphocytes, fibrocytes, and, last but not least, the NCC's all serve

---

[1] Beloussov LV. *The Dynamic Architecture of a Developing Organism*. Dordrecht, Netherlands: Kluwer Academic Publishers, 1998.

as go-betweens between tissue differentiation and the final outcome or function of tissues.

In this chapter, we will explore the NCC's, which can be considered as pluripotent cells that have the potential to differentiate in neurons, mesenchyme, or endocrine types of cells (eg, chromaffin cells of the adrenal glands). The NCC's link various types of cell and tissue differentiation within a brief lapse of time—that is, they are active for only a short period, before neural tube closure and during its closure.

It is as if NCC's transport space and time quanta of a very specific inductive area, such as rhombomeres, to anatomically separated target layers that need to integrate these messages to differentiate and find their definitive specification. In a certain sense, NCC's could be considered as the ideal expedient of the developing CNS for articulating with and informing specific target tissues during a well-defined lapse of time.

NCC's inform tissues that are linked by mesenchymal articulations that express their ambivalent properties throughout an individual's lifetime. The best examples are the tissues that differentiate from the circumpharyngeal crest. As those tissues continue their development, they eventually constitute the myofascial tract of all subhyoidal muscles and fascial layers that link the heart to the base of the skull. Several protagonists participate in the process that forms this pathway to the base of the heart. Part of this history will be elucidated in the following paragraphs.

2.2 Neural crest: the fourth germ layer of the body

Two types of cells seem to be important in the structuration and spatial organization of the body:
- Mesenchymal cells, which originate from the ectoderm germ layer during early embryonic life and act as an articulating system during tissular and structural organizations and adaptations (inductive processes).
- Neural crest cells, which originate from the previously specified neurectoderm layer, leaving the neural tube mostly at its dorsal end (with some exceptions, such as the seventh cranial nerve) and organizing distant articulations between different functions of the body.

A remarkable fact may be that both types of cells possess an astonishing capacity of migration and mobility. They play important roles in the transmission of information at cellular and tissular levels.

The neural crest produces a vast array of structures in the embryo. Its importance is such that it is sometimes called *the fourth germ layer of the body*. [1] Many structural and functional transformations of cells and tissues are induced during this proliferation phase of neural crest cells (➤ Fig. 2.1):
- The connective tissue and muscular walls of the large vessels arising from the aortic arch are informed by cells of neural crest origin. [2] Interfe-

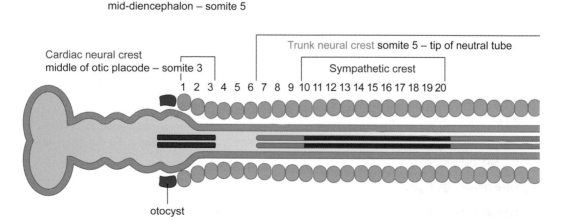

Cranial neural crest
mid-diencephalon – somite 5

Trunk neural crest somite 5 – tip of neutral tube

Cardiac neural crest
middle of otic placode – somite 3

Sympathetic crest

1 2 3 4 5 6 7 8 9 10 11 12 13 14 15 16 17 18 19 20

otocyst

Fig. 2.1 Distribution of cranial, cardiac, and trunk neural crest cells along the developing neural tube

rence with the embryonic neural crest leads to anomalies at this site, such as translocation of the two principal arterial trunks.

- The NCC's support the development of the endothelium of the aortic cross, they form the aortic-pulmonary septum, and they provide support to the muscular walls of the tunica media in all the arteries branching off from the aortic cross.
- The NCC's interfere with the pharyngeal endoderm and support the maturation of the thymus, parathyroid glands, and thyroid gland. [3–5]
- It is intriguing that the intrinsic neurons of the gut are of neural crest origin. [6] In view of the high rate of gut-related immune disorders found in strong left-handers, it could be assumed that there exists a relationship between the time of migration of these cells to the gut and the maturation of particular areas of the cortex.
- The asymmetry of scoliosis is suggestive of unilateral failure of dorsal root formation and, therefore, of unilateral disordered neural crest migration. [7]
- The migrations of NCC's are determined by both intrinsic properties of the migrating cells and features of the external environment encountered by the migrating cells. [8] (➤ Fig. 2.2)

Mechanical events play an evident role in the development and migration of NCC's. Neural tube closure in the cervical area (closure 1) begins at the location of the bend in the embryo, which tends to draw the two folds of the neural crest together. This fact suggests, according to Jacobson and Tam (1982), that the bend may *mechanically* assist closure in the cervical region. There is a second closure (closure 2), which overlies the bend—the cranial flexure. The direction of this flexure tends to spread the neural folds apart, probably acting as an impediment to closure. Each major region of the forming neural tube may have a unique combination of mechanisms providing the force for elevation of the neural folds. [9]

Some of the dynamic properties of these cells can be understood by studying the principles of biodynamic and biokinetic mechanisms that build structure, form, and spaces in the developing body, as mentioned by Blechschmidt and Gasser. [10] Every structure, form, and function is built upon three dynamical properties of cells and tissue:

- electrophysiological exchange
- nourishing currents (eg, transmembranous electrical potential, thermal gradient, space)
- degradation of currents (inducing cell apoptosis).

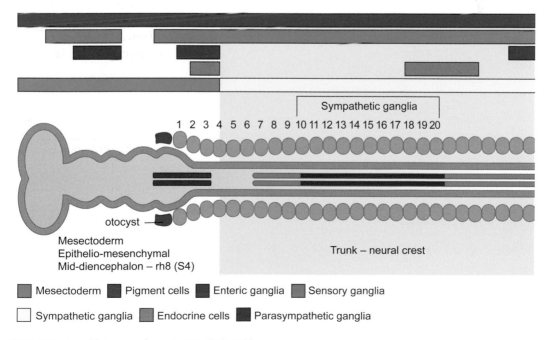

otocyst

Mesectoderm
Epithelio-mesenchymal
Mid-diencephalon – rh8 (S4)

Sympathetic ganglia
1 2 3 4 5 6 7 8 9 10 11 12 13 14 15 16 17 18 19 20

Trunk – neural crest

■ Mesectoderm ■ Pigment cells ■ Enteric ganglia ■ Sensory ganglia

□ Sympathetic ganglia ■ Endocrine cells ■ Parasympathetic ganglia

Fig. 2.2 Overlap of fate maps of neural crest cells (NCC's)

It can be stated that the molecular and electrophysiological equilibrium determine the exchange of metabolites and the tonality (tension, elasticity, and mobility) of tissue. The polarization of the body allows for the possibility of exchange (metabolism), coaptation (strength), and mobility (movement). The polarization principle can also be seen as the fertilized ovum consumes oxygen and glucose. During this process, the fertilized ovum changes its form from circular to ovoid (the zona pellucida), creating a restraining area in its middle part and preparing for mitosis (➤ Fig. 2.3).

The cell can be considered as a metabolic field exhibiting movements of particles inside and outside. These movements not only sustain metabolic exchange but are also composing parts of the tensegrity mechanics that are found in every tissue of the body. [11–19]

At the end of the second week, the zygote starts a nidation process into the endometrium. Nutritional absorption of metabolites in contact with the uterus epithelial covering is initiated. The metabolic field of the zygote produces cohesion of cells near the endometrium, pulling them together and driving out waste products on the opposite pole of the blastomeres. In this way, a first cavity is created—the ventral coeloma (or ventral coelom). (➤ Fig. 2.4) On the dorsal side, a first amniotic cavity becomes visible, and it is soon replaced by a definitive cavity—the dorsal coeloma (or dorsal coelom).

During this phase, a restriction area is also created, by the interaction of the cytotrophoblast and the dorsal coeloma. This restriction zone will later become the insertion area for the allantois on the caudal part of the embryo. The function of this articulation area during the late blastocyst phase is the exchange of oxygen and glucose. *Apparently, the site of nidation is*

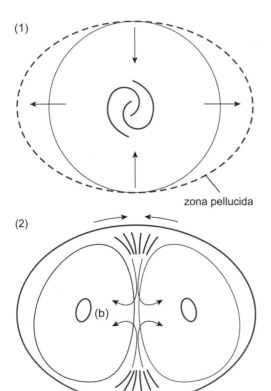

Neural Crest

(1) Fertilized ovum (zygote) consumes oxygen and glucose (altered after Blechschmidt and Gasser)

(2) Zygote cleaves to form blastomeres
(a) restraining area and nutritive area
(b) adhesive forces organized by electrolytic exchange

Fig. 2.3 Epithelio-mesenchymal transitions of cells could be due to intrinsic properties of the blastomeres and early differentiating cells, altering cell membrane tension and composition via electrolytic exchange.

(1)

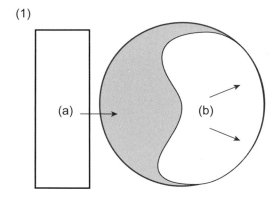

Neural Crest

(1)
(a) nutritional absorption of metabolytes in contact with uterus epithelial covering
(b) additional nutritive intercellular movements in the ventral coeloma and ventral ectoderm

(2)
dropping of epiblast cells that form hypoblast cells and rearrange Heuser`s membrane

(2)

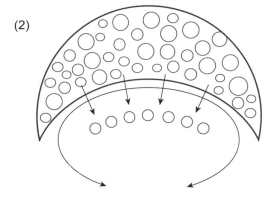

Fig. 2.4 Intrinsic metabolic processes support cell migration and differentiation.

determined by the degree of concentration of oxygen and glucose, which could be dependent upon the degree of vascularization of the endometrium.

During the second week, there are two other important developments:

• The formation of vacuoles in the syncytiotrophoblast by its interaction with the primitive epiblast cells, preparing vascularization of the later placenta. This process is called exotrophe (destruction of maternal cells and release of substances that provide the zygote and embryo with nutrients) (➤ Fig. 2.5).

• Further compression of the cell aggregation in the second week, to create an entocyst disc. During the increase in compression, the disc becomes bilaminar. The thicker layer adjacent to the dorsal endoblast chamber is the ectoderm; the thinner layer adjacent to the blastocoel is the endoderm. Between these layers, a basement membrane forms.

The surface area and thickness of the zygote increase primarily in the region where it is in contact with nutrients (ie, near the discal pole). Due to the position of the zygote on a large source of nutrients, it becomes lens-shaped. The main growth occurs in the region of the equator (the restriction area). This zone becomes particularly cellular. Metabolic movements, vacuolization of tissue, and the orientation of the zygote as a trajectorial structure are paired processes. In other words, the trajectorial structures show the constructive formative function of the zygote as a fundamental feature of its metabolism.

Blechschmidt and Gasser conclude that, based on their observations, *mesoblast formation, from the kinetic viewpoint, results from the unequal growth rate of the ectoblast and endoblast.* The intercellular substances in the mesoblast (the early inner tissue) do not stagnate but flow along the neighboring limiting tissue. This metabolic movement is called a *parmeation.* (➤ Fig. 2.5) This parmeation is important for

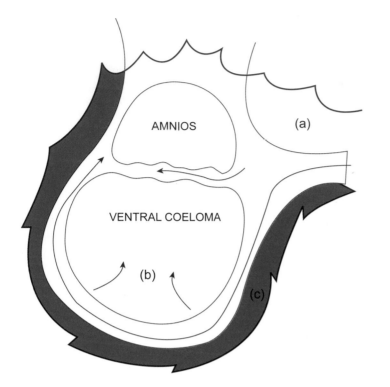

Neural Crest

(a) parmeation
(b) vitelline circulation
(c) extracoelomic mesoblast

Fig. 2.5 Vacuolization is a supporting process for cell migration and creation of trophic currents.

giving rise to the later vascular circulation. In regard to the entocyst disc, one can note a convex bending toward the dorsal blastema fluid of the ectoderm, due to the gradually increasing resistance of its basement membrane, thereby forming an expansion dome. *In this way, the basement membrane contributes to the differentiation of cells.*

During the initial differentiation processes (in the third week), the disc becomes S-shaped, and the yolk sac becomes an appendage of the disc. This structure is comparable to the anlage (a structure at the earliest stage of development) of an endocrine gland that gradually loses its vitelline duct (➤ Fig. 2.6).

The entocyst disc establishes a divergent growth in its cranial part and a convergent growth in its caudal part during the S-shape evolution. The basement membrane beneath these ectoderm cells does not expand. As a result, a depression forms in the ectoderm (the impansion pit). *The formation of positive and negative reliefs (the expansion dome and impansion pit, respectively) in the entocyst disc is the initial event that outlines the origin of the embryo.*

During the third week, one can observe eccentric movements of the ectoderm around the mechanical restraining point of Hensen's node, with more important growth in the cranial part of the entocyst disc. A restraining area is also found in the circumference of the disc, where the marginal mesoderm changes the form of the ovoid surface with a waist-like area around the middle part.

Due to the different growth rate of the ectoblast (epiblast) cells and endoblast (hypoblast) cells, an inner tissue similar in structure and origin to that of the mesoblast arises between these two layers. *Inner tissue develops when the surfaces of two adjacent, limiting tissues grow at different rates.* Mesenchymal and mesodermal tissue constitute a well-defined articulation area between two opposite tissue layers and growth rates. The mesodermal tissue could be considered as a storage place for growth differentiation and growth rate. It could also be considered as the first anlage of the extracellular matrix, which could concentrate a large amount of trophic factors, growth factors, and fibroblasts. These molecules

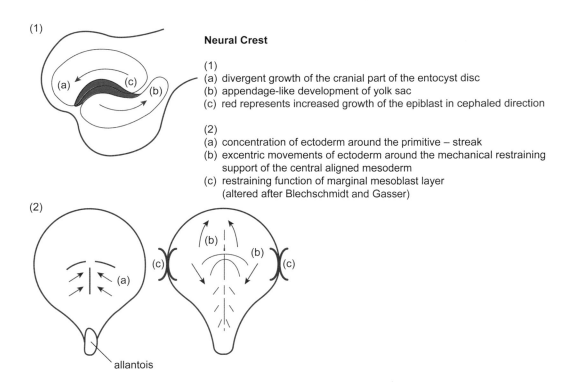

Neural Crest

(1)
(a) divergent growth of the cranial part of the entocyst disc
(b) appendage-like development of yolk sac
(c) red represents increased growth of the epiblast in cephaled direction

(2)
(a) concentration of ectoderm around the primitive – streak
(b) excentric movements of ectoderm around the mechanical restraining
    support of the central aligned mesoderm
(c) restraining function of marginal mesoblast layer
    (altered after Blechschmidt and Gasser)

Fig. 2.6 Cell migration and compaction processes support form transition and structuration of different subtypes of tissue.

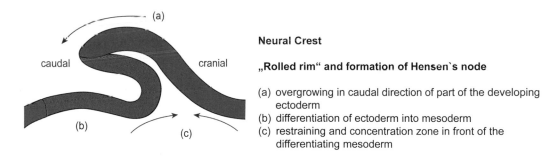

Neural Crest

„Rolled rim" and formation of Hensen`s node

(a) overgrowing in caudal direction of part of the developing
    ectoderm
(b) differentiation of ectoderm into mesoderm
(c) restraining and concentration zone in front of the
    differentiating mesoderm

Fig. 2.7 Formation of notochord process and, subsequently, of Hensen's node

could favor further development and differentiation of cells and tissues, dependent upon the time schedules of their specification during particular episodes of embryogenesis and organogenesis. Perhaps this function ultimately sustains other functions (eg, biomechanical) during adult life.

The area of the impansion is eventually overlapped by the caudal border of the expansion dome as a result of the unequal growth of the ectoderm layer. The so-called "rolled rim" area is referred to, in static terms, as Hensen's node (➤ Fig. 2.7). The formative

function of this differentiation is the development of the axial (notochordal) process. This process is the most important part of the next developmental movements in the embryo, by guiding cranial differentiation (between prechordal and parachordal plates) and by serving as an induction pole for most other cellular differentiations.

The movements of cells through the primitive knot and primitive streak are accompanied by major changes in their structure and organization. As the epiblast cells enter the primitive streak, the cells elonga-

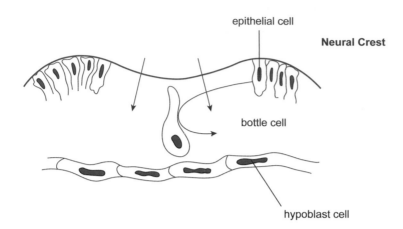

epithelial cell

Neural Crest

bottle cell

hypoblast cell

Fig. 2.8 Formation of Hensen's node and migration of cells that underwent epithelio-mesenchymal transition and migrate as bottle cells. An identical process can be supposed for migration of NCC's.

te and take on a characteristic morphology that has led to their being called "*bottle cells*." Within the primitive groove, these bottle cells assume the morphology and characteristics of mesenchymal cells, which are able to migrate as individual cells (➤ Fig. 2.8). The cells spread between epiblast and hypoblast to form the embryonic mesoderm. The epiblast cells facilitate their movements by producing hyaluronic acid. The spread of mesodermal cells away from the primitive streak (or the equivalent structure) depends on the presence of fibronectin, which is associated with the basal lamina beneath the epiblast.

At the level of the notochord, the neurenteric canal forms. This channel's precise function is unknown, though it provides temporary continuity between the amniotic cavity and the yolk sac. *It may provide the only direct communication that ever exists between these two cavities.* Later communication between the amnion and endocoelom is assured by excretions of the fetus into the amniotic cavity, as well as by fetal drinking of this same amniotic fluid (starting at approximately the 50th day). [20]

The notochordal process functions as a primitive inductor for the anlage of the nervous system. Retinoic acid is produced at Hensen's node, functioning as a morphogenetic signaling molecule for the transformation of ectoblast cells into nervous system cells. Activin and TGF-β2 seem to play important roles in the induction of the mesoderm. *It further seems evident from experimental studies on avian embryos that the primary hypoblast exerts an inductive and morphogenetic influence on the overlying epiblast.*

The ectoderm, overlying the notochordal process, transforms into an elongated patch of thickened epithelial cells, called the neural plate. The whole transformation is orientated upon the prechordal, or prochordal, plate tissue. The notochordal process exerts a resistance against the ectoderm, causing its growth to become retarded. The axial process prompts the arising of the neural groove, and—as a consequence of its origin—the formation of the dorsal bulges (➤ Fig. 2.9).

The medial slope of the dorsal bulges greatly thickens, forming the epithelial anlage of the nervous system, while the lateral slope becomes relatively thin, forming the anlage of the body wall of the cranial, cervical, and trunk regions. One can note a para-epithelial supply of nutrients originating laterally from the chorionic cavity, as well as a metabolic exchange between the amniotic cavity and endocoelomic cavity, in a one-direction flux toward the developing neurectodermal tissue. This tissue is not a neural tissue in the true sense. Rather, it can be considered as an epithelial tissue with a polarized metabolic activity. In this way, the ectoderm layer may be considered as *a one-way polarized metabolic field* that releases catabolites on its free surface and assimilates substances on the side covered by mesoderm. [10]

Fluids in the interior of the mesoderm are sites of biomechanical pressure. Likewise, the cell-limiting membranes are sites of biomechanical stress. This is the way the laterally paired aortae are built in the lateral mesoderm anlage at the sites of para-epithelial nutrient supply (starting during the third week).

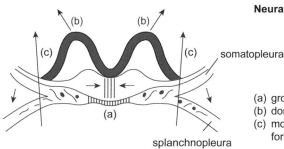

Neural Crest

somatopleura

(a) growth resistance of notochord
(b) dorsal bulging of neural plate, forming neural groove
(c) movements of nutrients from ventral to neural pole, forming a one-way polarized metabolic field

splanchnopleura

Fig. 2.9 Appearance of dorsal bulges at the neural groove localizes most of the interference between neural ectoderm and epiectoderm. Reciprocal induction processes determine the differentiation of most of the NCC's of the early embryo.

The somite development closely follows the unequally growing ectoderm. Dorsal paired branches of arteries and veins segment the somite vesicles. The mesenchyme slowly grows together with the blood vessels under segmentation furrows, forming the segmentation septa. *The somitic capsule probably arises as a result of sliding movements, with the somites playing an important role in the orientation of the migration of the neural crest cells.* In other words, the dorsally placed dermatome produces chondroitin sulfate proteoglycans, thereby creating a physical barrier against the dorsally migrating neural crest cells. The formation of an individual somite involves the transformation of cells with a mesenchymal morphology to a sphere of epithelial cells within the paraxial mesoderm. Neural crest cells migrate through the intersomitic spaces, penetrating only the rostral half of each somite.

This process is related to the segmentation pattern of the dorsal root ganglia and the sympathetic ganglia.[2] [21] If one considers the development of neural crests, one can remark that the crests appear to be tangentially pulled from the dorsolateral side of the neural tube. These cell aggregations exist only dorsolaterally and move tangentially away from the central nervous system.

This cell movement can be explained entirely by the kinetics of the surrounding structures. As the neural tube grows, the tensile strength of the meninx and the restraining function of the dorsal intersegmental vessels pull the neural crest cells out of the neural tube. The pull of the primitive dura acts tangentially on the dorsal part of the neural tube, thereby initiating the formation of neural crests. [9, 22] The fluid pressure between endomeninx and ectomeninx also plays an important physical role in the orientation of the spinal ganglia and the reunion of dorsal root and ventral root trajectory. [10] (➤ Fig. 2.10)

The same process can be demonstrated for the growing cortex. As the cerebral surface enlarges in three dimensions, the cell processes align in dimensions that are parallel as well as perpendicular to the anlage of the pia mater. Neurons migrate within the white matter, which exhibits a *fluxion field* for all descending neurites. The appositional growth of the cortex occurs in a direction opposite from the basal ganglia.

The migration of the neurons is structured by glial cells that organize around the ventricles (peri-ependymal layer) in an ascending pattern, forming columnar radial units. [23] *These glial cells are partly of the same cell lineage as the neural crest cells.*

- The first glial cells of the primitive cortex are usually astroglial cells. These cells can transform in a transient way into radial glial cells. Radial glial cells are typically thin, filamentous, stretched bipolar cells that cover the distance between the ventricular zone and the pial side of the subcortical/cortical plate. They branch in these marginal zones and form the final connection sites with the pial membrane. *The radial glial cells are used as a*

2 Le Dourain N. "Les cellules de la crête neurale migrent dans les espaces intersomitiques et pénètrent exclusivement dans la moitié rostrale de chaque somite à l'exclusion de sa moitié caudale. Ce processus rend compte de la segmentation des ganglions rachidiens et sympathiques." [21]

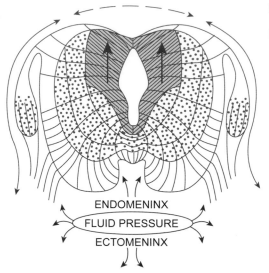

Neural Crest

Nervous System

ENDOMENINX
FLUID PRESSURE
ECTOMENINX

Fig. 2.10 Fluid pressure at the level of the ventral endomeninx/ectomeninx and traction at the level of the dorsal ectomeninx guide the movement of migratory cells in a ventral direction.

kind of rope ladder by neurons during their migration out of the ventricular germinal zone in the direction of the cortical plate and their fixation to it. They codetermine the distribution and approximate location of the migrating neurons and the pattern established by transcription genes and growth factors. Neuronal migration over these rope ladders is supported and guided by complex molecular processes, such as cell membrane adhesion processes and signal detection by ligands. (➤ Fig. 2.11) The migrating neurons establish specialized contacts with these radial glial cells during their displacement. These contacts are broken after reaching their target by unknown mechanisms. The radial glial cells transform into astroglial cells after the end of the neuronal migration process.

- These morphological changes of the radial glial cells could be influenced by the postmitotic neurons and regulated by an unknown factor that is not membrane-bounded.
- Experiments have provided evidence that the Cajal-Retzius cells play a regulatory role in the morphology of the radial glial cells.
- The Cajal-Retzius cells probably also influence the direction in which the migratory process evolves.
- Further evidence exists that Cajal-Retzius cells are the main source of the reelin protein, which is

needed for correct cell-to-cell interactions during the development of the cortex.
- Most of the migrated neurons during this early period disappear and are no longer in place at the adult stage (as a result of pruning/apoptosis). The cause of this apoptosis process is not well understood. It's possible that the Cajal-Retzius cells disturb synaptogenesis by their overactivity. The production of glutamate could create an increased calcium flux and, thereby, organize accelerated cell death.
- The dendrites of the Cajal-Retzius cells display intimate contact with the overlying mesenchyme and are necessary for regionalizing neuronal migration and nidation. When these contacts are disturbed, deficits in corticalization appear.
- Early disturbance of radial glial cell formation can be elicited by additional factors, notably alcohol abuse. [24]
- Cajal-Retzius cells display minimal electrical activity resembling neuronal activity. They could be important in establishing coherence during the phase-locking of different neuronal "trains" in cortical field activation.

The restraining function of the ectomeninx at the base of the brain offers a growth resistance for the basal part of the cortex. It has become obvious that intense, eccentric, antibasal growth of the cerebral

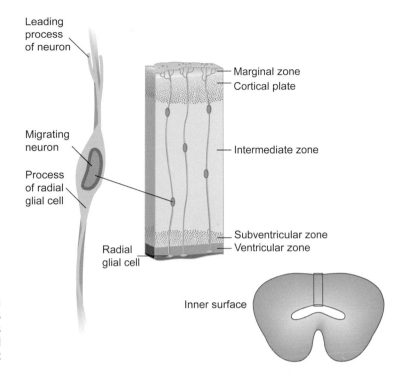

Fig. 2.11 Cell migration—such as the migration of neurocytes upon a radial glial ladder—is based on mechanical, amoeboid processes, as well as the intrinsic properties of the cells.

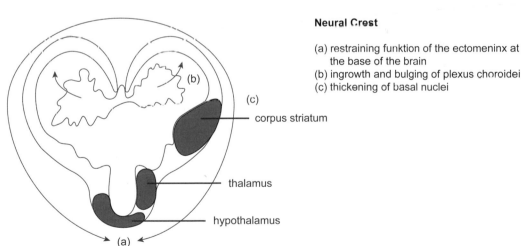

Neural Crest

(a) restraining funktion of the ectomeninx at the base of the brain
(b) ingrowth and bulging of plexus choroidei
(c) thickening of basal nuclei

Fig. 2.12 Compression and topography of groups of neurons and mesenchymal cells are due, in part, to compressive forces of the enveloping tissues.

hemispheres is an important prerequisite for the high degree of differentiation of the human cortex. The endomeninx (the anlage of the pia mater) lies adjacent to the brain wall and contains many blood vessels. As the ventricle wall attempts to expand by each vascular pulsation, the thin, weak areas of the hemispheres (medial walls) protrude in the direction of least resistance (ie, toward the ventricles). (➤ Fig. 2.12) Some areas of the brain grow convexly, in such a way that they gradually come to

2

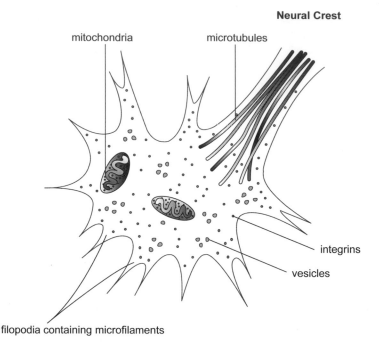

Neural Crest

Fig. 2.13 Cell elements participating in neurotaxis

abut against one another. The ectomeninx (anlage of the dura mater) in the areas of abutment becomes stronger, forming restraining bands, or dural girdles. The dural girdles appear to curb brain growth to such a degree that the brain bulges in the areas between the bands.

It is clear that cell mobility and migration are dependent upon the adjacent cell layers and the surrounding tissues, which serve as an exploration field for definite function.

It is argued by both B. Freeman and E. Blechschmidt that the general impression of cell motion and migration could be an incomplete representation of what really happens during cell emplacement and differentiation.[3] These mobile properties could be supported by general bending and torquing movements of the embryo as a whole. Cells would be displaced by changes of form and field in the growing embryo as they adapt to altered spatial relationships. The immobile point of reference could be situated at the apex of

the chorda, functioning as a point of zero motion around which the sequences of displacement and organization of the embryo are organized.

Another important aspect of morphological transformation is that much of the functional and anatomical differentiation is determined by the fields to which the differentiating, migrating structures are attracted. The molecular and chemical gradients of that field, together with the location at any given moment of embryological development, play important informative roles in the determination and specification of forms and functions.

If we consider the patterns and mechanisms of neurite outgrowth, we notice that a growth cone caps an actively elongating neurite. In vitro and in vivo studies of living nerves have shown that *the morphology of an active growth cone is in a constant state of flux, with filopodia regularly extending and retracting as if testing the local environment.* This phenomenon cannot be considered only as a mechanical event, but also as a molecular and biochemical exchange between the neurite and its environment. The growth cones contain numerous cytoplasmic organelles and large quantities of actin microfilaments that determine the form and function of the filopodia. Growth co-

[3] Freeman B. The active migration of germ cells in the embryos of mice and men is a myth. *Reproduction.* 2003;125:635-643.

nes can respond to concentration gradients of diffusible substances (eg, neurite growth factor) and to weak local electrical fields. They can also respond to fixed physical or chemical cues from the microenvironment immediately surrounding them. (➤ Fig. 2.13)

Neural crest cells break from the neural plate or neural tube by changing their shape and properties from those of typical neuro-epithelial cells to those of mesenchymal cells. [25] Migration of NCC's in the head region begins before closure of the neural tube; in the trunk region, it occurs after closure. During their migration, these cells lose the function of their cell adhesion molecules (CAM's); after migration, the CAMs become functional again. Migration is sustained by the activities of fibronectin, laminin, and collagen IV. Chondroitin sulfate, produced by the dorsal part of the somite, inhibits dorsal migration of the NCC's.

Part of the NCC programming seems to occur before the cells leave the neural tube. Additional developmental potential is determined by the environment through which the cells migrate and into which they finally settle. Transplantation experiments in vivo have revealed evidence of the effects of the embryo's environment upon the progressive determination of NCC development during and at the end of migration. Recent research has attempted to identify the environmental factors that are responsible for these influences. Endothelin 3 (EDN3) could play a major role in the development of the two main derivatives of the neural crest lineage— the melanocytes and the cells of the enteric nerve system.[4] [9]

There is increasing evidence of a correlation between the time of emigration of NCC's from the neural tube and their developmental potential. NCC's that begin to migrate early in the process have the potential to differentiate into many different types of cells. NCC's that begin to migrate later in the process are capable of forming only derivatives characteristic of more dorsal locations (eg, spinal ganglia), but not sympathetic neurons or adrenal medullar cells. The last NCC's to leave the neural tube are restricted to the most dorsal pathway of migration and can form only pigment cells.

Neural crest cells from the trunk differentiate into sympathetic neurons that produce norepinephrine as a transmitter. Neural crest cells from the cranial region give rise to parasympathetic neurons, which produce acetylcholine. However, it is clear that the fates of NCC's are not irreversibly fixed along a single pathway. Three main migratory pathways for trunk NCC's can be noted (➤ Fig. 2.14):

- A ventral pathway between the somites and the neural tube, continuing under the ventromedial surface and reaching the dorsal aorta; *this is the sympathoadrenal lineage.*
- A ventrolateral pathway that leads into the anterior halves of the somites; these cells form the segmentally arranged *sensory ganglia.*
- A dorsolateral pathway between the ectoderm and the somites; these cells form the *pigment cells (melanocytes).*

Neurite outgrowth and functional organization is mainly orientated as a strip of condensed cells forming a so-called *ectodermal ring* on the surface of the developing embryo (➤ Fig. 2.15). Migration and functional organization of neural crest cells are orientated by the different placodes in the head region (eg, optic, otic, nasal placodes), resulting in: 1) the route of the fifth cranial nerve (trigeminus nerve) and 2) the circumpharyngeal crest orientated along the route of the twelfth cranial nerve (hypoglossal nerve), also called the hypoglossal cord. [26] In the trunk region, the main route is organized by the sympathoadrenal lineage, as previously mentioned.

The hindbrain shows a segmental nature during the first eight embryonic weeks. This segmentation into rhombomeres is parallel to the development of the somitomeres in the same region. The cranial nerve nucleus distribution indicates a regular pattern of origin, at every two rhombomeres. A relationship between homeobox gene (ie, Hox gene) expression and fundamental patterning processes within the central nervous system, as well as other components of the body, is widely assumed. Because cellular differentiation begins in the hindbrain, the segmental

---

[4] Des expériences de transplantation in vivo ont mis en évidence l'effet de l'environnement embryonnaire sur la détermination progressive des cellules de crête neurale au cours et à la fin de leur migration. Les recherches actuelles tendent à identifier les facteurs de l'environnement qui sont responsables de ces influences sur la crête neurale. L'endothéline 3 (EDN3) joue un rôle crucial dans le développement de deux dérivés importants de la crête neurale; les mélanocytes et le système nerveux entérique."[9]

Development of neural tube
NCC: Neural Crest Cells: dorsalizing

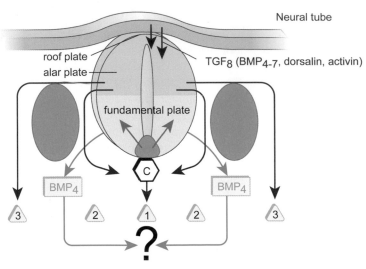

1. Ventral pathway: sympatho-adrenal lineage
2. Ventro lateral pathway: sensory ganglia
3. Dorso lateral pathway: pigment cells

Fig. 2.14 The three main migratory pathways of trunk NCC's are oriented by space and time and related events.

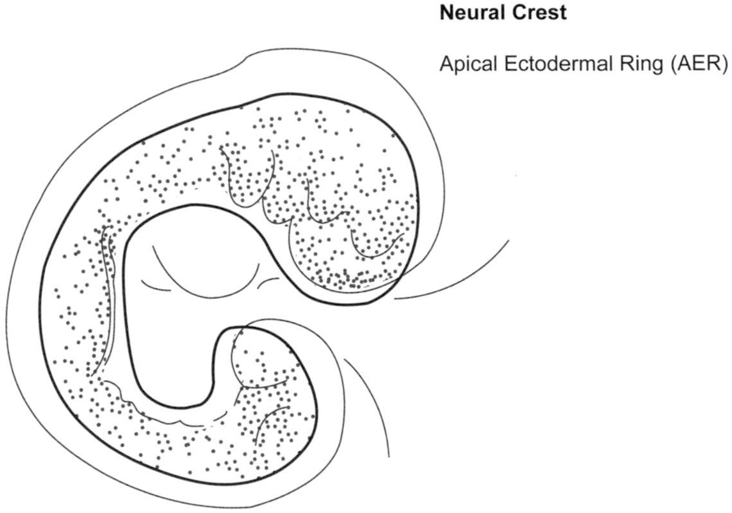

Neural Crest

Apical Ectodermal Ring (AER)

Fig. 2.15 The apical ectodermal ring forms a compressed border of epiectodermal cells that are capable of organizing some placodes and limb anlagen.

nature of the neural tube again becomes evident when cellular behavior is considered. The correspondence between the rhombomeres of the developing brain and other structures of the cranial and pharyngeal arch region is remarkable. In the region of the hindbrain, several sets of placodes, developing in concert with the local neural crest, participate in the formation of the sensory ganglia in the cranial nerves.

Considering the cell lineages in the central nervous system, we can find *a final articulation* between the mature neuron, on the one hand, and a large differentiation of the glial progenitor cell, on the other hand, effectuated by the microglial cell. These cell types are mesodermally derived immigrant cells, serving a phagocytic function after brain damage. Microglial cells are not found in the developing brain until it is penetrated by blood vessels. They display an electrical pattern in association with the neural tissue they support in the adult brain.

A unique characteristic of neural crest cells is their ability to move long distances. The intercellular spaces enlarged by hydrated glycosaminoglycans, the large amount of fibronectin in the basal membranes and other intercellular structures, and the presence of other lectins serve as guidelines for the pathways of NCC's.[5] [27]

2.3 Patterning: an interaction between a core link and lateralizing impulses

The organization of form and structure is dependent upon specific events that start during the early stages of embryogenesis. Many of these events could be defined as principles for structure formation, organization, and differentiation.

Without delving too much into the molecular field of cell organization, one could note a progressive differentiation of cells and tissue around a central axis and a more or less equilibrated lateralization process. This lateralization process seems related to a core link that continuously changes its quality of interaction with surrounding tissues, depending upon the ventralizing and dorsalizing impulses of various effector genes.

During the early blastomere stage of development, one can find a polarization of cells into an animal pole (the more animated, mobile pole) and a vegetative pole (the less active pole). This polarizati-

on of the blastomeres organizes a trophic field and a constructive field.

The midline organization during the polarization of the blastomeres is the first, "invisible" axis of organization in embryo development. It is probable not only that the blastomeres react upon cell-cell interactions and cell-cytoplasm interactions, but that the surrounding environmental cues are influential in blastomere organization. The electrical field and polarity of the environment of the zygote could play major roles in the organization of blastomeres, including their first functional alignment.

Most research into the axial cranial-caudal development of embryonic organization has concentrated on the study of gene-transcriptor protein interactions (eg, Hox genes, Hom genes). However, it would be interesting to study how an already organized blastomere field changes its axial patterning when the blastomeres are placed in an altered electrical field, inducing an altered electrical or electromagnetic polarity. In this test case, one might discover if the genes are proactive or responsive.

What are the successive steps in midline formation?

The first step, as we previously mentioned, is the invisible midline organization during the blastomere stage, which is dependent upon cell polarization and cell-environment interaction.

The second midline formation appears during gastrulation. During this stage, one can note a sinking of the epithelial ectodermal cells, which organise a visible midline, the linea primitiva. The ectodermal cells apparently first form a primitive line and a central knot before they begin to grow in an ascending, appositional way to form the neural bulges. It seems as if these cells delegate part of their constructive potency to an intermediate tissue for constructing a definite midline for the whole body plan. This body plan is preceded by an axial gene mapping, as we previously mentioned.

Mesenchymal "bottle cells" condense ventrally around the linea primitiva and also migrate cranially and laterally between the ectoblast and endoblast cell layers. These cells will form a wide variety of tissues, ranging from cartilage to vessel walls. The "director" that governs the midline function at this stage of development is the anterior extremity of the chorda dorsalis, the chordal process. It is like the

---

[5] *"Ein besonderes gemeinsames Merkmal der Neuralleisten-Zellen ist ihre Fähigkeit, zum Teil über erhebliche Strecken zu wandern. Die durch hydratisierte Glycosaminoglycane erweiterten Interzellularräume sowie der hohe Gehalt an Fibronectin in den Basalmembranen und anderen Interzellularstrukturen sind – neben anderen Lectinen – Leitstrukturen für den Wanderungsweg dieser Zellen."* [27]

conductor of the central row orchestra, guiding the expansive movements of mesenchymal cells and precursor neurons.

The ectoderm cell layer that will form the neurectoderm gives off dorsalizing and ventralizing signals (eg, dorsalin, BMP4) that induce dorsal or ventral development of cells in the trilayer organization of the embryonic disc. The cells interact and differentiate to establish definite ventral and dorsal midlines. The ventral midline is represented by the chorda dorsalis, which develops into the dense, structural midline. The dorsal midline differentiates into the neural tube, representing a more fluid electrical midline.

During this phase of cell differentiation and organization, there is an ascending appositional proliferation of neurons. This ascending migratory pathway around the ependymal canal is characteristic for brain development, as well as for medullar development. At the final stage of formation of the neural bulges, some neural precursor cells at the edge of the bulges interact with the overlying epidermal cells and differentiate into neural crest cells. These NCC's further differentiate and migrate according to patterning based on time/space information that is partly inherent to their intrinsic coding and partly dependent upon environmental cues. They wander between the somites in a ventral direction and colonise different sites of the body on the basis of time and place of segregation.

Some of the cells follow cranial pathways (eg, trigeminal strands, hypoglossal cord), others follow and form the sympatho-adrenal lineage, and still others migrate more laterally and superficially (eg, melanocytes). It appears as if the cells are conditioned to reach the anterior and central sites of the body. During this migration, they use the mesenchymal substrate, which is organized like a tridimensional patchwork of connective tissue that connects the neurectoderm with the developing endodermal and mesodermal organ primordiums.

The NCC's display a tendency to articulate the ventral and dorsal midlines (ie,chorda and neural tube) with the anterior and central alignment of the body. Part of this pathway is patterned by ectomesenchymal and epithelio-mesenchymal cell interaction, such as epithelio-mesenchymal transition and mesencyhmal-epithelial transition. It seems logical

to accept that the dorsal and ventral midlines contribute to the formation of an anterior localized target tissue that will condense around anterior central alignment.

It further seems reasonable to assume that a third midline is prepared, the ultimate function of which is to contribute to hematopoietic, endocrine, and immune adaptive cell transformations that respond to continuously changing internal and environmental information. During the complete embryonic and fetal developmental staging, one can note that this anterior midline is progressively compressed in a dorsal-lateral-ventral direction and in a cranial-caudal direction. That means that the cells around this anterior midline are crowded by compressive impulses generated from the dorsal-ventral midline function. It is reasonable to suppose that part of the adaptive capacity of the body is concentrated in tissue substrates that preserve a potency to differentiate into specialised cells when needed (eg, the thymus gland, thyroid gland, sternal hematopoietic tissue, and germ cell layers of the urogenital apparatus) (➤ Fig. 2.16).

Besides the cranial-caudal patterning, one can note an almost simultaneous lateralizing impulse from the primitive midline. It has been established that a nodal flux (flow) on the ventral side of the embryonic disc organizes movement of the coelomic fluid in a preferentially left-side direction. This nodal flow is generated by the ciliated cells at the ventral side of the primitive line, especially at Hensen's node. This flow pattern facilitates the migration of morphogenetic proteins toward the left side of the midline. Meanwhile, the morphogenes with a right-side tendency seem to be inhibited.

This patterning by the nodal flow is likely supported by mesenchymal pathways that facilitate migration of other mesenchymal or neural crest cells during later stages of development. The pathways also could facilitate inductive processes that occur through paracrine signalling. One could suppose that mesenchymal migration is prepared by the nodal flow of fluids at the ventral coelom. The neural crest cells can then use these mesenchymal fields for their own migratory patterning. Certain molecular compounds, such as laminin and fibronectin, facilitate the migration.

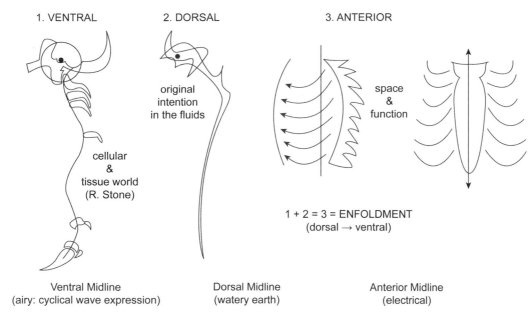

1. VENTRAL

2. DORSAL

3. ANTERIOR

original
intention
in the fluids

space
&
function

cellular
&
tissue world
(R. Stone)

1 + 2 = 3 = ENFOLDMENT
(dorsal → ventral)

Ventral Midline
(airy: cyclical wave expression)

Dorsal Midline
(watery earth)

Anterior Midline
(electrical)

Fig. 2.16 Orientation and organization of the different midlines commonly accepted in the osteopathic nomenclature

An identical nodal flow is described at the dorsal side of the embryonic disc, where Hensen's node also seems to be the organizer. This is a strong indicator that the neural tube is informed by the lateralizing coding of the genetic mapping. The lateralization of the flow organizes a generalized left-sided Ca^2 flux, which equally influences the patterning of the brain, heart, and intestines ($\succ$ Fig. 2.17).

The NCC migratory pathways in the autonomous nervous system could represent the go-between for the electrical patterning of laterality between the ectoderm and endoderm anlagen. One has only to study the anatomy and function of the parasympathetic and sympathetic nervous systems to understand that these functions are also more or less lateralized, and that, at most of their final synapses, they present an intermingled pattern. Thus, the mesenchymal cells and connective tissue could represent the go-between for the mechanical and metabolic relationship between the ectoderm and endoderm anlagen.

Preliminary conclusions concerning this chapter on neural crest and mesenchymal patterning could be stated as follows:

- The polarity of the blastomere field creates the possibility to establish a primitive midline that

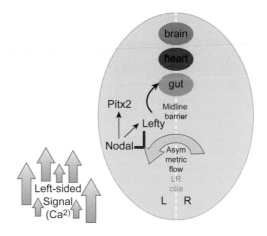

Fig. 2.17 The lateralization process starts by left-sided Ca^2 signalling, influenced by the Pitx2 transcription factor, at the level of the embryonic disc.

serves as a reference for further cell migration and structuration.
- The primitive midline, in turn, supports and organizes a lateralizing tendency of the coelomic and amniotic fluids that supports the lateralizing tendency of the genetic mapping.
- The interconnection between ectoderm and endoderm anlagen is referential to an organizing mid-

line and, at the same time, functional by a laterali-zing tendency of the connecting field established by the mesenchymal and neural crest pathways.

- Both functions (neural and metabolic) are con-nected by a well-established electrical and me-chanical anatomy supported by the autonomous nervous system and the connective mesenchymal fields between the two substrates.

Finally, one could propose that the midline supports the lateralizing tendency of structuration of the ex-change field (metabolic, mechanical, vascular), and that the relative stability of the lateralized fields sup-ports the integrity of the midline function.

REFERENCES

[1] Carlson BM. Human Embryology and Developmental Biology. Philadelphia, PA: Mosby, 1994.

[2] Bockman DE, Kirby ML. Dependence of thymus deve-lopment on derivatives of the neural crest. Science. 1984;223(4635):498–500.

[3] Kirby ML, Waldo K. Role of neural crest in congenital heart disease. Circulation. 1990;82(2):332–340.

[4] Kurutani SC, Kirby ML. Initial migration and distributi-on of the cardiac neural crest in the avian embryo: an introduction to the concept of the circumpharyngeal crest. Am J Anat. 1991;191(3): 215–227.

[5] Rosenquist TH, et al. Origin and propagation of elas-togenesis in the developing cardiovascular system. Anat Rec. 1988;221(4):860–871.

[6] Geschwind N, Galaburda AM. Cerebral Lateralization. Biological Mechanisms, Associations and Pathology. A Bradford Book. Cambridge, MA: MIT Press, 1987:165.

[7] Cilluffo JM, et al. Idiopathic ("congenital") spinal arachnoid diverticula. Clinical diagnosis and surgical results. Mayo Clin Proc. 1981;56(2):93–101.

[8] Ziller C, et al. Contrôle génétique et épigénétique du développement de la crête neurale. Bull Assoc Anat. 1998;82(259):46.

[9] Emmanouil-Nikoloussi EN, et al. Anterior neural tube malformations induced after all-trans retinoic acid administration in white rat embryos. Morphologie. 2000;84(264):4–11.

[10] Blechschmidt E, Gasser RF. Biokinetics and Biodyna-mics of Human Differentiation. Springfield, IL: Charles Thomas Publishers, 1978.

[11] Ingber DE, et al. Cellular tensegrity: exploring how mechanical changes in the cytoskeleton regulate cell growth, migration, and tissue pattern during morpho-genesis. Int Rev Cytol. 1994;150:173–224.

[12] Ingber DE. Cellular tensegrity: defining new rules of biological design that govern the cytoskeleton. J Cell Sci. 1993;104(Pt 3):613–627.

[13] Stamenovic D, et al. A microstructural approach to cytoskeletal mechanics based on tensegrity. J Theor Biol. 1996;181(2):125–136.

[14] Pienta KJ, Coffey DS. Cellular harmonic information transfer through a tissue tensegrity-matrix system. Med Hypotheses. 1991;34(1):88–95.

[15] Gumbiner BM. Cell adhesion: the molecular basis of tissue architecture and morphogenesis. Cell. 1996;84(3):345–357.

[16] Wang N, et al. Mechanotransduction across the cell surface and through the cytoskeleton. Science. 1993;260(5111):1124–1127.

[17] Ingber DE. Tensegrity: the architectural basis of cellular mechantransduction. Ann Rev Physiol. 1997;59:575–599.

[18] Ingber DE. Integrins as mechanochemical transducers. Curr Opin Cell Biol. 1991;3(5):841–848.

[19] Guan JL, Chen HC. Signal transduction in cell-matrix interactions. Int Rev Cytol. 1996;168:81–121.

[20] Nebot-Cegarra J, et al. L'embryon humain est-il capab-le d'ingérer le liquide amniotique. Bull Assoc Anat. 1996;80(251):54.

[21] Le Douarin NM. La crête neurale. Une structure pluri-potente de l'embryon vertébré. Bull Assoc Anat. 1996;80(251):13.

[22] Witkop CJ, et al. Optic and otic neurological abnorma-lities in oculocutaneous and ocular albinism. Birth Defects Orig Artic Ser. 1982;18(6):299–316.

[23] Rakic P. Specification of cerebral cortical areas. Science. 1988;241(4862):170–176.

[24] Supèr H. Cajal-Retziuscellen in de ontwikkeling van de cerebrale schors. Neuropraxis. 1999;1:14–20.

[25] Monteagudo M, et al. Observation des premières cellules de la crête neurale dans l'espace mésoder-mique dorsal adjacent au tube neural. Bull Assoc Anat. 1996;80(251):52.

[26] O'Rahilly R, Müller F. The early development of the hypoglossal nerve and occipital somites in staged human embryos. Am J Anat. 1984;169(3):237–257.

[27] Hinrichsen KV. Human Embryologie. Heidelberg, Germany: Springer Verlag, 1990:126–127.

CHAPTER

3

About pediatrics

3.1 Interaction between the cell and the extracellular matrix (ECM)

The first steps in morphogenesis can be considered as cell-to-cell interactions needed to create an ambient substrate in which the cells can transform and exchange information. Most of the authors on embryology mention the importance of the cellular environment in fully expressing the genetic potential of the cell.[1]

Morphogenesis can be considered as a differentiation and integration process of polyvalent patterns of function and structure. There exists a feedback system between the fundamental substance—the extracellular matrix (ECM)—and differentiation antigens produced by differentiating cells in their glycocalyx. These antigens activate regulator genes (homeotic genes), which possess the consensus sequences for particular stretches of DNA. The homeobox genes code for the transcription factors that bind to the DNA.

We may suggest that all cell-to-cell and cell-to-environment interactions are "sequence-linked" processes from the beginning. They enable exchange and differentiation. The more complex these exchanges become, the more important will be the role of the fundamental substance (ECM) in permitting the transformation and migration of the ectoderm and endoderm cells of the basic germ layers. The

ECM provides a three-dimensional network of collagen in which ectoderm and endoderm cells transform into mesenchymal cells, creating in this way a specific time-space related network.

This could mean that the ECM contains differently informed time-space relationships dependent upon specific moments of important cell transformations and migrations. Mechanically or chemically activating a part of the ECM could evoke a particular moment of evolutionary progression in tissue-organ maturation. Cell movements during these evolutionary periods are largely based on contractile properties of the mesenchymal cell itself (actin and myosin filaments) as well as on chemical gradients of the environment (chemotactic movements, or haptotaxis). The fluidity of the tissue is guaranteed by secretion of hyaluronic acid, which, at the same time, permits cell migration and inhibits further cell differentiation.

Estrogen- and progesterone-receptors, located on mesenchymal fibroblasts, control early mesenchymal differentiation: estrogen increases hyaluronic acid production, and progesterone inhibits it. [1] The same determining function of estrogen and progesterone antagonism is found in the early differentiation of the brain and the determination of the embryo's sex, as stated by Galaburda and Geschwind. [2]

A great deal of cell differentiation seems determined by pressure and traction forces exerted on the developing tissues. Piezo-and pyroelectric effects alter tissue viscoelasticity and are interpreted as differentiation impulses by the cells. The tissue integrates a considerable part of the mechanical information as stress, and it will try to restore its original biological state as well as possible. If these efforts are not successful, the tissue will try to restore its initial state by integrating the impulses as part of its mechanical property or by differentiation processes. That is the reason why each impulse has to be considered as a

---

[1] Heine states: *"Die Entwicklung einer Zelle zu bestimmter genetischer Expressivität, Form und Funktion in einem mehrzelligen Organismus wird durch die Beziehungen zu ihrer Umgebung bestimmt. Die wechselseitigen Beziehungen zwischen Zelle und Grundsubstanz sind bereits Voraussetzung zur Entwicklung eines Keimes."* Heine H. Lehrbuch der Biologischen Medizin. Auflage 2. Stuttgart, Germany: Hippokrates, 1997:168.

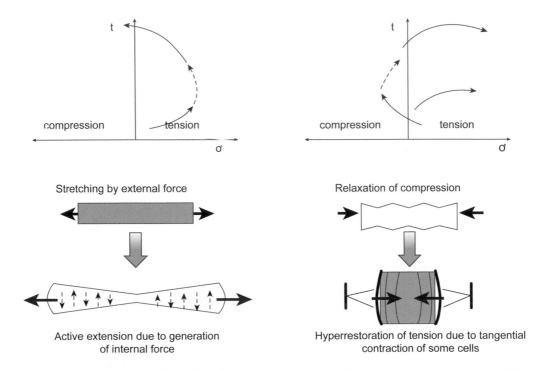

Fig. 3.1 Each stress on a tissue is followed by an increase in tension, succeeded by a relaxation/compression phase, which could be considered as tissue "overshooting."

transformer of the original space/time relationship of the biological system.[2]

Conversely, one could consider the tissue as a transforming and integrative unit that initially expresses a kind of "protest" against each change of its integrity, before finally integrating the impulse as a new part of its developmental memory. The mechanism for restoring this mechanical integrity of the tissue has been defined by L.V. Beloussov as a "stress hyperrestoration response" (➤ Fig. 3.1).[3]

We could suggest that throughout the processes of cell differentiation/maturation and birth, there is an equilibrated cooperation between intrinsic genetic and extrinsic chemical and mechanical inputs, allowing the embryo to acquire its definitive structure and form. *This is an important consideration for the osteopathic approach during the prenatal and perinatal period, when the informing hand of the osteopath, through touch, traction, and pressure, could activate or direct tissue physiology.* Apparently all dynamic processes are based upon biochemical, molecular coding sustained by mechanical parameters—even the descent and expulsion of the fetus. *The hand of the osteopath could be a fulcrum in establishing the correct environment for all chemical and mechanical events to take place in an equilibrated manner and/or for supporting and reactivating tissue/cell-integrated memory during morphogenetic and morphodynamic developmental stages.*

The biochemical mechanisms implicated in the initiation of parturition are still not well understood. Are these mechanisms dependent upon signals of the fetus, or are they induced by the mother?

Prostaglandins seem to be the most probable actors for the induction of the birth process. The quantity of prostaglandins increases in the amniotic fluid, the blood, and the maternal urine. In cell culture, prostaglandin E2 (PGE2) has been shown to increase the extensibility of the tissue of the cervix, as has PGF2α.

[2] Bacques P. *L'homme moléculaire et son psychisme.* Paris, France: Maloine, 1974.

[3] Beloussov LV. *The Dynamic Architecture of the Development of Organisms.* Dordrecht, Netherlands: Kluwer Academic Publishers, 1998.

Lefèvre [3] proposes three hypotheses:
- The placenta itself may possess the capability of secreting a neuropeptide normally secreted by the hypothalamus. This neuropeptide, called corticotropin-releasing hormone (CRH), stimulates the hypothalamo-hypophyseal-adrenal axis. Its action results in the secretion of adrenocorticotropic hormone (ACTH). This same ACTH is also found in the human placenta, where it may influence the fetus by increasing the production of fetal glucocorticoids. In this way, it interferes with fetal maturation. CRH also stimulates the secretion of prostaglandins, an important chemical signal for the induction of labor.
- The cytokines may be produced by the maternal macrophages and lymphocytes, responding to bacterial aggression and inducing an increased production of prostaglandins by the fetal membranes (according to experiments done in vitro). Recently, it has been discovered that the tissues of the uterus release cytokines without any underlying infection. Interleukin 1 (IL-1) and tumor necrosis factor (TNF) are the most preponderant of these cytokines.
- A third hypothesis is more interesting for the osteopath, because it underlines the important role of the amniotic fluid as a "translator" between mother and fetus. This fluid is in intimate contact with the fetal membranes and is a principal site of production of prostaglandins. A substance secreted by the fetal kidney—similar to epidermal growth factor (EGF) and released in the amniotic fluid—seems capable of stimulating the secretion of PGE2 by the amnion in vitro. Another factor possessing the same properties is platelet activating factor (PAF), secreted by the fetal lungs.

It is interesting to observe how the fetus produces certain quantities of pro-urine (an osmotic exchange product) and urine, which are secreted in the amniotic fluid, first by simple transmembranous exchange and later by excretion through the urinary tract. These excretions determine volume and quality of the amniotic fluid. We could state that the fetus uses this fluid as a transducer between the internal environment and the external environment. Part of the fluid is integrated at the level of the developing tongue papillae, where they serve as a stimulus for further maturation of the gustatory nerve tract and

the primitive endoderm (especially the foregut). At this level, we find the most fundamental substance composing the epithelium of the mucosal layer of the rhino- and oropharynx. A smaller quantity of fluid is also ingested at the lung level, where it probably sustains lung bud maturation.

A more biophysical or biomechanical hypothesis could be that the pressure-volume relationship between the amniotic sac and the amniotic fluid has two functions:
- Fluid pressure upon the enveloping membranes may exert a kind of shear force that stimulates the membranes to secrete some peptides and tissue hormones necessary for normal physiology.
- The volume of amniotic fluid seems to be an indispensable factor to safeguard the fetus against excessive direct pressure.[4] However, this same fluid could serve to guide the fetus into the pelvic girdle of the gravid during the early birth process.

Either too much or too little amniotic fluid could impede the harmonious descent and orientation of the fetus into the birth canal. The quantity of amniotic fluid could be a determining factor in translating the force of the uterine contractions during labor pains. The fluid quantity may also be the greatest origin of compression of the fetus, especially of the fetal skull.

It could be that slight compression and fascial release exerted by the hands of the osteopath upon the uterus of the gravid during fetal descent suffice to coordinate the normal physiology of the early birth process.

It is likely that compressive forces are not only elementary for guiding a normal descent of the fetus, but they also seem indispensable for the normal orientation of the head in the birth canal (ie, right or left occipital orientation).

Even more important is the probability that the asymmetrical compressive field surrounding the fetus plays an important role in favoring a more prevalent right or left dominance of the cortex. Related to this, we find biomechanical and psychomotor

---

4 A Potter syndrome may be the best example of what can go wrong without the mechanical role of amniotic fluid as a buffer against excessive pressure of the uterus and surrounding membranes upon the fetus. The characteristic "Pott's face" is one of the particularities found with oligohydramnios.

patterns more or less expressed in the functional adaptation of the youngster.

Galaburda and Geschwind [2] and other authors provide us with the following observations:

- All living things find themselves in an atmosphere of asymmetrical physical forces that are the result of Earth's geological characteristics and the planet's position in the universe. Sunlight, magnetic forces, and gravitational forces probably all play important roles in creating asymmetrical patterns of form and function in plants and animals, including human beings. A pattern of asymmetrical forces acts on the human brain in its passage through the birth canal. Although most infants exit in the left anterior (LOA) position, three less frequent birth positions also occur. Some authors have argued that the infant's position in the birth canal leads to asymmetrical forces on the brain that later affect cerebral dominance. A strong relationship has been demonstrated between birth position and later handedness, with ROA infants having a much higher frequency of left-handedness than LOA infants.
- The position of the head must depend either on asymmetry in the birth canal or on asymmetry in the skull. When the head rotates into the LOA position, the longest diameter of the head lays in the axis of the birth canal, and the narrowest diameter is at right angles to this axis. In other words, the head is in the position that offers the least resistance to movement.
- As the uterus contracts, the head will move into this position of least resistance. The fact that the forces of uterine contraction are powerful and that the head is readily molded by these forces need not negate this possibility, because even a small deviation from symmetry in the head might lead to an asymmetrical effect in the cortex.

Habib M, et al [4] mention a study by Galaburda and Levitsky in which they investigated the asymmetric aspect of the right and left planum temporale, a cortical area hidden in the Sylvian fissure. They found that in about two out of three cases, this area was more developed at the left hemisphere. This site includes the Wernicke area, known to integrate linguistic information, a somewhat specialized function of the left hemisphere (though the right hemisphere is also partly involved in the linguistic outcome). The authors concluded that this asymmetry displays a functional feature and is specific for almost the whole brain.

The asymmetric pattern of the planum is present at birth, offering evidence that morphological aspects are closely related to neuropsychological properties. Trophic factors, such as estrogen and testosterone, and also structural factors are capable of influencing the normal development of neurons and their migration at specific moments of development. It is probable that trophic and structural factors, which are active during the period of neuronal migration (sixth month of gestation), both favor a functional, atypical lateralization pattern.

3.2 Osteopathy and the birth process

For the osteopath, it is clear that the process of birth is one of the most critical periods in life, determining a great deal of the definitive harmonious relationship between structure and function.

The cranium is submitted to great physical stress during its passage through the birth canal. As previously mentioned [4] asymmetry is partly a normal expression of life processes and partly a determinant of dysfunction in the lateralization pattern. The rotational pattern by which the cranium descends in the birth canal is determined by the shape of the pelvic girdle of the mother. Both the innominate lines and the sacral promontory serve as reference places by which the young skull is "impressed."

Most adult skulls still manifest some impressions and strain patterns representing the pressure exerted by the promontory. These patterns suggest the integrated route the skull took to descend in the little pelvis. It is reasonable to suppose that the skull impressions not only have to be considered as possible lesion-inducing events, but that they probably also incorporate some innate functional patterns from the maternal pelvic girdle.

I would like to hypothesize that part of the pattern found in the young skull should be considered as a functional expression of a primary transmission of maternal information into the cartilaginous structure of the young infant. A functional pattern could be diagnosed as the facility of the skull to mold more easily in one favored dimension than in another. This molding occurs without the presence of lesions of synchondrosis sphenobasilaris (SSB) or sutural or intraosseous lesions.

In my opinion, every skull possesses such an early-impressed pattern. Studying this pattern could reveal much about the prenatal biomechanical relationship between mother and child. It is also probable that these structural impressions inform the immature brain and continue to do so later in life, by sustaining psychomotor development or even psycho-emotional reaction patterns.

If we accept W.G. Sutherland's statement that "as the twig is bent, so the tree will grow," then it is not so strange to think that an early mechanical impression could determine early and later, induced reaction patterns of the brain. H.I. Magoun wrote the following:*"The skull of the infant is highly vulnerable to the forces of labor. Its physiologic lack of development, the pliability necessary for the birth process, the abundance of cartilaginous and membranous tissue which later ossifies, the possible disproportion between the passage and the passenger, the extensive molding which often occurs, the distortion of pre-osseous elements, the adaptive deformities which are so rapidly included in the postnatal development and ossification – all these militate against the achievement of normal structure and function in the unit mechanism of the body."* [5]

Sutherland was probably one of the first osteopathic physicians to underline the importance of a normal labor process in establishing a healthy relationship between skull and brain: [6]

"Osseous tissue is held together by membrane and cartilage and so arranged that the infant head can adapt to the maternal passageway. The parietal bones can fold over the frontal and occiput and between the temporals for an easier passage into the world. Can anyone doubt that there is movement at that period? The bones do not have articular mobility but they do have movement. The normal cranium in infants and children provides for growth but you do not find significant articular gears forming until the age of ten, except a little here and there.

The articulation between the condyles of the occiput and the facets of the atlas is the one established joint at birth. These occipito-antlantoidal joints are ligamentous articular mechanisms. Otherwise, there are no articular surfaces because there are no joints with "gears" at birth. The formation of articular gears for articular movement between the bones, at the sutures, of the human cranium becomes more established around the seventh to ninth years of life, or even later. "Even following a normal delivery, there is a situation that calls for attention. The baby's head has adapted mechanically to the passageway during birth. When the baby cries and inhales air, aided by atmospheric pressure, the cry is usually vigorous, a special cry, with or without a spank on the sacrum. The process fluctuates the cerebrospinal fluid. Then the membranes go to work and pull the bones into position.
"Recall that the bones in the cranial base form in a cartilaginous matrix are in parts at birth. The four parts of the occiput surround the foramen magnum. The sphenoid is in three parts at birth, and the temporal bones are in three parts. Consider the possibility of disarrangement among the parts as well as between the bones themselves under the various mechanical events of birth. Then visualize the growth of the cranial base during infancy. Do you see that the slow motion of growth may be a factor that is active in the problems resulting from the early patterns that persist?"

These words of Sutherland indicate that structure is not completed until the age of 10. Many other observations suggest the continuing sharing of mutual information between brain and skull until puberty has ended.

The growth of the infant skull depends largely upon the growth of the brain. This organ is quite immature at birth and comparatively late in acquiring blood vessels. However, all the nerve cells seem to be present at birth and, if severely injured, will not regenerate. Although some neoneurogenesis (development of new nerve fibers) has been discovered at certain places of the adult brain (eg, hippocampus, entorhinal cortex), the question remains regarding how far these new neurons can accomplish regeneration to counterbalance extensive nerve destruction.

These considerations underline the importance of the process of birth as the ultimate factor orientating later mental and psychomotor skills of the young infant. A normal process of birth requires numerous well-coordinated factors and events. During a normal birth, the left parietal, being posterior, meets resistance from the promontory of the sacrum. Being retarded in this manner, its medial border slips under the edge of the right, or anterior, parietal, which is descending more rapidly behind the symphysis pubis. Meanwhile, cerebrospinal fluid and blood have been discharged from the cranium, lessening its volume to some extent, and the occiput and frontals have telescoped beneath the parietals, further decreasing the head size.

To bring the sagittal suture anteroposteriorly, as well as to straighten the neck, rotation takes place when the head reaches the resistance of the anal gutter. The base of the occiput then slips beneath the symphysis pubis.

There is some molding of the fetal skull during the last month of pregnancy for the impending passage, though this consists mainly of the moderate overriding and compression previously described. This normally corrects itself in the infant with a few days of crying, which balloons out the perimeter of the skull, and suckling, which flexes the sphenobasilar sychondrosis via the vomer and normalizes the pull of the intracranial membranes. [7]

The molding process in the last month of pregnancy caused by uterus contractions is one of the most important factors stimulating the elastic behavior of the immature sutures. This prepares the skull for its to later "opening" after the birth process, induced by the primary cries of the baby. Of course, contractions that last excessively long can contribute to compression of the skull or deformation into a lesion. Even the amount of surrounding amniotic fluid plays an important role in transmitting the contractions of the uterus muscle upon the skull.

Magoun mentions heredity, maternal health, use of drugs, abnormal pelvis, prematurity, abnormal presentation, abnormal forces, abnormal delivery, abnormal oxygen and hemorrhage as factors that determine perinatal lesion mechanics. [7] Skull deformation and malformation are well defined by other authors. [8, 9]

- *Deformation* refers to an alteration in the shape of a part that has differentiated in a normal manner. In most cases, the cause of the altered form is fetal crowding or intrauterine molding. Most deformations are engendered in the third trimester, a time when the fetus grows rapidly in comparison to the volume of amniotic fluid and uterine space in which it gestates.
- *Malformation* refers to an intrinsic arrest in normal embryogenesis.
- *Disruption* refers to the destruction of an anatomic part that had previously differentiated normally. Hemi- or craniofacial microsomia also have a disruptive pathogenesis: interruption of blood flow through ischemia or hemorrhage in the developing fetal face leads to a focal deficit in facial growth.
- *Craniostenosis,* in some cases, seems to be due to premature apposition of the calvarial plates at the cranial sutures. [10]
- *Plagiocephaly* is a term that refers to a flattening of the cranial contour, usually in the posterior parietal region. This may lead to a prominence of the contralateral parietal region and the ipsilateral prominence of the upper face and cheek [8].
- *Orbital malformations*—such as hyperteloric orbits, shallow orbits with consequent proptosis, and asymmetric orbits—can all place mechanical stresses on the eye(s) in one or more positions. Less frequent etiologies for strabismus in patients with these anomalies include paresis of the third, fourth, or sixth cranial nerves and alteration in the number and structure of extraocular muscles. Interestingly, operative intervention directed at the orbital malformation may have little effect on strabismus. Although correcting the orbit may reduce some of the stress, long-standing strabismus often leads to secondary muscular changes, such as hypertrophy or contracture, that resist realignment. [8, 11]

Remarkably, most prenatal skull lesions are indicative of interference resulting from mechanical stresses, genetic predisposition, and vascular ischemic causes. The pathological pattern is probably coordinated by the same structure that also organizes and integrates normal skull development, namely the dural membrane. Albright and Byrd [10] mention that the determinants of cranial shape include the rate and directions of brain growth, the form of the cranial base itself, and the insertions of the dura on the cranial base. The dura is both the periosteum of the calvaria and the guiding tissue in the morphogenesis of the calvaria and its sutures. An altered cranial contour is typically due to primary abnormality of the cranial base.

V. Fryman[5] mentions that the first action in pediatric craniosacral therapy is to examine if the cranial base is free and able to express a normal degree of flexion/extension. If not, one may admit that the cranial base has been compressed and cannot exhibit normal vitality.

Many of the "deficits" that the cranium will express later in life can be hidden in the still supple and adaptive reciprocal tension membrane organization. Only obvious defects, such as major cranial deformations, may be noticed by the medical doctor. Subtle dysfunctions, such as slight strabismus or deficits in sucking, will not be associated by the medical doctor with possible underlying cranial lesions. Thus, these dysfunctions are completely dependent upon the cranial diagnosis made by the well-trained hand of the osteopath.

The prenatal and perinatal periods are critical in organizing the "mechanical behavior" of the skull and its related functions. Months or years later, some neurosensorial, behavioral, or even orthopedic deficits will manifest themselves as late expressions of the early-induced lesions. Dental caries, thumb sucking, and orthodontic malformations may all be consequences of malalignment of cranial components.

- Thumb sucking occurs in 13% to 45% of all children under the age of four years. The most common manifestations of thumb sucking are protruded and intruded upper incisors, intruded and retruded lower incisors, anterior displacement of the maxilla, anterior open bite, and posterior crossbite.

- Dental caries (tooth decay) continues to be a major disease, particularly in the child with craniofacial anomalies. It appears that dental caries is a multifactorial disease requiring the presence of a susceptible host, cariogenic microflora, and diet conducive to enamel demineralization. Dental caries is caused by anaerobic bacterial production of acid as a byproduct of carbohydrate metabolism. The salivary buffers are unable to neutralize the acid, which cannot diffuse out of the plaque surrounding the teeth. [8]

- Recurrent respiratory distress could be related to subtle craniofacial deformities or disturbances, which may be perinatally or congenitally organized.

- Trauma or buckling from disproportionate growth of skeletal facial structures is generally accepted as an explanation for the occurrence of septal (septum nasi) deviations, which are found most frequently in adult males. Evidence supports the view that these deviations can also result from parturition injuries sustained during rotation of the fetal head in the birth canal. Indeed, they are reported to be less frequent in cesarean deliveries than in vaginal births. A recent series of studies cited a 2% rate for septal deviations in neonates.

- Objective measurements prove that rapid maxillary expansion (a common orthodontic procedure), in addition to enlarging the upper dental arch, widens the piriform aperture and results in a marked and lasting increase in nasal patency.

- Chronic mouth breathing is widely regarded as an important etiological factor in developmental abnormalities of dentition and facial structure in children. [12]

Congestion of the mucosa of the nose and naso/oropharynx can be either the cause or the result of cranial deformations that express themselves in the area of the viscerocranium. A close relationship can be found here between the functioning of the gut and the cranium. Epithelium similar to the gut epithelium extends into the mouth, even into the eustachian tube, and this tissue displays the same features of immune response wherever it is located. One could wonder if, in early life, localized immune reactions in the mouth or larynx are synchronized expressions of more distant suffering in the gut. Could it be a kind of trial and error of the immature lymphoid tissue to adapt and organize upon a wide diversity of pathogens?

The postnatal period seems to be an extremely critical time for the harmonious development of the young skull. Certain areas, such as the fonticuli and some synchondroses, play crucial roles in early life to spread different mechanical stimuli in the ossifying cranium. Sucking, biting, upright positioning of

5 Fryman V, Moschalenko Y. Conference; 2001; Utrecht, Netherlands.

the head, and eye movements are all dissipated in the sutures and osseous trabeculae of the skull. The greatest part of these force lines will, in later life, determine the ability of the skull to adapt to exogenous mechanical, neurosensorial, and emotional needs. Scoliosis capitis [13] is, for the osteopath, a well-known manifestation of strains upon the skull base, especially upon the occiput.

Many ossification areas display specific, critical periods of ossification. Cranial normalization of distorted areas should have happened before these critical periods. A short overview about these periods of ossification, as described by Hauser G. and De Stefano G.F. [14], should increase the osteopath's awareness of the importance of interfering with the processes before these times:

Ossification of the synchondroses and fontanels of the skull.
- Condylar parts of the occiput:
  The anterior parts of the occipital condyles are formed from the basilar part; the other part of the condyle belongs mainly to the lateral part (exoccipital). The anterior intraoccipital synchondrosis, which separates these two parts, begins to ossify at the age of six and is fused after the age of eight.
- The fonticuli:
  The anterior fontanel is the largest of the fontanels in the late fetal stages, and it closes at about the middle of the second year of postnatal life. It has a quadrangular kite-shaped form. The fonticulus anterolateralis (sphenoidal fontanel, or pterion) is obliterated within two or three weeks after birth.
- The posterior median fontanel is triangular and closes at about the time of birth or shortly thereafter. If there are ossicles at bregma or lambda, they often reflect the shape of those two fontanels. The fonticulus posterolateralis (mastoid fontanel, or asterion) closes during the first postnatal year.
- The sutures:
  The coronal, sagittal, and lambdoid sutures permit minimal movements of the skull bones during delivery and are areas along which further bone growth occurs. Thus, they contribute to the change in size and shape of the skull.

Sutural structures are genetically determined, but environmental factors (forces derived from cranial growth, brain growth, or other processes) are required for the manifestation and development of the qualities of the structure (eg, manifestation of lingulae and inner abutment plate). Onset of obliteration generally takes place between the ages of 30 and 40 on the inner surface and about 10 years later externally. Lack of intrinsic motion of these particular regions can be an important indicator of early mechanical stresses upon the skull, and it may also be the key event for switching from normal physiology into pathology of the brain.

Fluid exchanges between the different meningeal spaces and the intracranial and extracranial venous plexuses can determine a great deal of early appearing intracranial pathology. The osseous compressed compartments can play particularly crucial roles in the organization of altered electrical fields in specific brain areas and in the orientation of peripheral musculoskeletal axes that control biomechanical patterns of the body.

3.3 The natural birth process, a mechanical pattern that articulates internal and external forces

The expulsion process during birth is an interesting event for the observing eye of the osteopath.[6] Life, in its extra-uterine dimension, apparently receives its final form during the expulsion phase. The young body is subjected to such mechanical forces as compression, rotation, and flexion/extension—without any long-lasting deformation or impairment of physiology. One could state that these patterns stimulate normal physiology. Many of these mechanical strains are likely integrated in the cartilaginous and fascial structures of the young body. Perhaps they

---

[6] It was A. Chila in one of his conferences in Belgium (Namur/Wepion, 2001) who stated that a good osteopath has to do three things: "See, look and ... perceive." [15]

can be used in the learning processes of the body as referential or integrative patterns.

The baby is expulsed in a more or less spinning pattern that facilitates and supports the birth process. Coinciding with this pattern, it could also be observed that life and the matter structured around it are rotational expressions of energy rather than linear processes. That means that most of the structures in the body are conceived and organized in a spiraling pattern.

The spiral organization of the body is apparently the best adaptation for integrating and expressing the different physical laws of life. Gravity invites the body to exploit these spiral types of motion, though humans primarily express linearity in their motion patterns. *We could state that the linearity of motion in man is a result of the freedom the rotational pattern in the body's experiences.*

This rotational pattern molds the skull of the baby before and during birth. The skull is compressed inside the pelvic girdle of the mother, and the sacrum and promontory mark the skull before it is expulsed and decompressed. It is obvious that these influences force the elastic tissue of the skull to adapt to and integrate opposed forces in a gradually more structured and reactive organization.

Very often, the promontory stays inserted in the bony organization of the skull as a landmark of the birth process. When one slightly compresses the skull of a youngster or even an adult, the cranium may re-expose its original rotational pattern, showing a mechanical balance point. That is the point where the original rotation "waits" for a reorganization of its energy. Frequently, this anatomical landmark is localized in the posterior temporoparietal junction, near the asterion.

This point of compression could be conceived as one of the first points of balance in the young body. It often builds up a balance point in the rotational pattern of the skull, and it is able to accumulate perverted energy throughout life. It can become both the starting point and the endpoint of the energy exchange of the whole skull and of the body.

A second compressive force is established at the occipito-atlantoidal (OA) articulation at the moment of birth. This area is hyperextended against the symphysis pubis of the mother. Most cranial osteopaths believe that this movement of hyperextension

stretches the vital membranes of the skull and the spine to initiate the breathing pattern of the Tide—the vital impulse that activates all forms of cell motility. The long Tide becomes integrated in a well-defined direction and increasingly expresses its specific rhythmical pattern.

Also at the level of the OA articulation, the rotational pattern prevails. The head is already definitely impressed, and the fasciae passing through this level receive a preferential organization. The implicated forces in this early life period are very important for organizing the adaptive and integrative capabilities of the body.

W.G. Sutherland observed that, at birth, the OA articulation is the only genuine articulation of the core link. It seems self-evident that most of the keys for integration and adaptation to physical strains will be inserted in this area.

The rotational patterns in the body seem to be the best-adapted modes for integrating and reexpressing the mechanical vectors of energy in life. One can imagine that when these patterns are not sufficiently free—due to perinatal traumatism, for example—the integrative capacity of the body decreases.

The same is true for the capability to absorb traumatizing energy later in life. A bump or punch, for example, demonstrates linear progressions of energy that should normally be easily absorbed into the spinning pattern of the body. To be harmless for the body, linearity has to be as easily absorbed as rotational energy. Only when the implicated force becomes too powerful for the integrative capacity of the body will the rotational pattern express dysfunction. Part of the rotational organization will absorb a maximum amount of kinetic energy, but it will become unable to restore an outgoing linear pattern.

The shock can be transmitted in the osseous parts of the body, which contain well-adapted spiral bony lamellae for this kind of integration. But if the shock exceeds the absorption capacity of the bone, it is possible for the a-physiological shock wave to compress any articulation of the body. It is also possible that the shock ends up in the fluidic organization of the body. In that case, the body fluids will perpetuate the disturbing interference through altered patterns of fluid expansion and retraction in most of the fundamental tissues of the body.

The CSF, endolymph, perilymph, and the fluids of the camera bulbi and aqueous humor are privileged target sites where shock-energy can reside and alter fundamental physiology. There are multiple symptoms and consequences of this shock, including general fatigue, depression, nausea, dizziness, visual and auditory acuity changes, and such articulatory changes as arthritis. Fluids contained in the peritoneal cavity and pericardial sac are minimal in quantity, but they probably also undergo these perverting forces. In the long-term, the forces may install an insidious progressing pathological pattern.

As R. Becker[7] states, "the symptom ignores the cause."

The accumulation of shock-energy can be conceived of as a state of fibrillation of the concerned tissues or fluids. When this happens, the tissues or fluids start to emit a kind of stiffening of the rhythmical fluctuating expression of energy that sustains normal physiology in that region. The bone, the cartilaginous structures of the body (discs, menisci), and the fundamental substance (ECM) all seem to be adapted to convert these shock-waves into inoffensive and even functional rotational patterns. The accumulated energy can be prolonged in a functional rotational pattern if not too much rotational overload exists.

An interesting array of probabilities merge when one studies these integrative capacities of the body.

- Linearity (as an exogenous force) is integrated in the body as rotational capacity. It can reinforce or stabilize the intrinsic force of the body.
- When the implicated force is excessive, the body tries to perpetuate this expansion in the rotational organizations of the implicated region.
- When this capacity is insufficient, the external force becomes the organizer of the disturbed pattern. It starts acting as an energetic cyst or as a disturbing stillness in wavelike expression.
- Eventually, the body will lose its rotational potential and organize a linear motion pattern that predisposes it to trauma. The normal spinning patterns of the joints, as well as the integrative capa-

city of the supporting tissue and fluid, will be disabled and favor the development of pathology.

- The nonadapted linear movement expressed by the body can be compared to the linear movement of a car that no longer can navigate the curving of a bend.
- The integrated excess of shock is eventually reconstituted by the body as an outgoing linear force that impedes normal physiology.

3.4 The postnatal landmarks of maturation involved in establishing adult patterning of body physiology

The first question asked by the osteopath should be about the origin of the symptom presented by the patient. When the osteopath has to treat a newborn, he or she has to rely upon the information provided by the parent or upon the diagnosis provided by a pediatrician. In most cases, the disorders presented by babies and children are based on functional disorders, indicating the possibility for functional treatment (though some disorders may hide deeper origins of pathogenesis).

When there exists a direct relationship between pathology and symptoms (eg, trauma, pathogens, heredity), a clear diagnosis can be established, allowing medical doctors to develop a more or less effective program. In this option, scientific research, leading to appropriate methods of diagnosis and treatment, has invaluable importance. In addition, the osteopath has to know the semiological and clinical skills for making a proper diagnosis and, thereby, avoiding inappropriate treatment.

The efficiency and precision of diagnosing early disease or hereditary abnormalities are increasing and extending into the earliest prenatal period. Surgical procedures in utero are now considered a fascinating feature—and the future—of medical technology and knowledge. For certain other pathologies, such as crying, cramps, vomiting, sleep disorders, cognitive and behavioral disorders, and orthopedic imbalances of the locomotion system, practitioners of conventional medicine have somewhat more

---

7 Becker R. *Life in Motion*. Portland, OR: Stillness Press, 2001; *The Stillness of Life*. Stillness Press, 2000.

limited capabilities—and should be grateful to nature for supporting the healing process.

The main question that remains in pediatrics could be posed as follows:

What is healing in a process of constant transformation, in which each tissue of every developmental field or organ of the young body is constantly in search of balanced exchange and adaptive integration of stimuli?

Additional questions are:

To what extent are external (exogenous) stimuli effective in stimulating or altering the homeostatic potential of the baby, and are they necessary for informing the definitive adaptive tools of the developing organism?

Is it normal that some disturbing episodes occur during the most essential physiological phases of field organization, such as immunity, endocrinology, growth, psychomotor skills, and communication?

Could it be that these transitory episodes also organize some adaptive procedures in the homeostatic field of the body?

In the osteopathic approach to the baby, we can only support, or sustain, the self-healing potential of the infant. By this, I mean that it is very doubtful that an osteopath is actually treating a disease in an infant. Rather than treating a disease, it is more probable that the osteopath is supporting the healing, or adaptive, process that is hidden within the secret of the continuously adaptive patterning of young tissues. The osteopath is probably supporting the healing process by potentiating the biological power of the tissue in all of its physiological properties, necessary for restoring a state of health.

In an abstract way, one could propose that the osteopath tries to be in synchrony as closely as possible with the secret of the tissue, rather than with the baby itself. The only way for understanding the suffering of the baby through a manual approach is by being confident in understanding the laws of tissue (which are the laws of nature and health). The more the osteopath knows about the chronological and functional development of the organizing tissues of the body, including its cavities and maturation of organic function, the more he or she can relate some expression of the problem to a particular period of prenatal or postnatal development.

The tissue is transmitting time/space-related scales of biomolecular and biophysical functioning in the hands of the osteopath, who has to accurately recognize and register the density, direction, vitality, and location of that particular tissue at that particular time of suffering. The density of a structure can vary in its structural constitution, but it can also vary in its electrical or vibratory (frequency) level. All of these features can modify the perception and interpretation of the state of the tissue, suggesting different interpretations of the diagnosed disease.

The following table offers an impression of the different states of physico-physiological "density" of tissue that could alter the interpretation of physiology—states that the palpating hand has to synchronize. (➤ Table 3.1) The table shows that physiology is constantly balanced by at least three states of interference with the body's inner and outer environment.

The fields of the newborn are predestined, but they are not finished at birth. They remain rather chaotic and are capable of adapting to a multitude of stimuli. The osteopath needs to be aware that by "informing" the tissue too much or by being too powerful, he or she could disturb the adaptive fields of the baby, directing them into patterns of adaptation resembling states of disease.

When we examine the fields that are important during successive periods of child development and when we want to be correct in supporting the normal developmental patterns that establish health, then we need to carefully study the main fields of embryological and fetal development. Here, one can see three main embryological fields supporting each other in a linear manner (cell to cell, cell to tissue), and additional fields developing in a reciprocal manner. After birth, this order is respected throughout the development of the infant to the teenager state.

The biggest demander is the brain, which is constantly requiring more energy and oxygen. These demands can be quantified in measures of regional cerebral blood flow and oxygen supplementation. For these needs, the brain is dependent upon blood supply and the pressure/volume handling of the cardiovascular system, which is organized into an adult patterning immediately after birth. The brain relies upon proper oxygen uptake at the lungs, which remain immature until at least two to four years after birth (lung maturation/alveolar maturation)—and

3

Tab. 3.1 At least three states of physico-physiological density, or structure, could affect the palpatory interpretations made by the osteopath.

Solid state	Fluid state	Energetic state
Biopolymers	Extracellular fluid	Matrisomes
• PG/GAG • Structure proteins	Endothelial and organizing fluids	• Glycocalyx • Microadaptive EFE
Mesenchymal transit	Parmeation-permeation streams	Photon > EME > Radiance > EFE
Connective tissue	A/V/L fluids	Frequency field and phases
Membranes-fasciae-tendons	Cardiopulmonary/renal	• Microcrystalline • Neural wiring
• Dense structure • Muscle, bone, cartilage	Cardiovascular system	Central/peripheral/autonomic/enteric nervous systems
Organized matter	**Organized volume**	**Organized frequency**

Abbreviations: A/V/L, arterial/venous/lymphatic; EFE, electric field energy; EME, electromagnetic field energy; GAG, glycosaminoglycans; PG, proteoglycans.

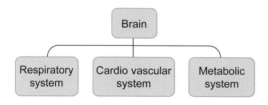

Fig. 3.2 The brain is associated with and governed by the three main systems of the body, guaranteeing basic homeostatic information exchange.

upon the digestive field for proper carbohydrate consumption. The digestive field also is immature at birth, requiring at least another seven years to be completely organized (development of the immune field of the endodermic tract).

In summary, the brain relies for its oxygen and energy demands upon two developmentally immature fields for at least the first decade of life. One could propose that immediately after the first decade, the immune field of the digestive tract becomes fully responsive and organized, allowing an adapted reciprocal exchange between the metabolic-cardio/respiratory-nervous webs.

If there is no structural or genetic dysfunction at birth, then one could propose that the fully outgrown brain relies upon the proper pumping of the heart, which interferes dynamically with the respiratory and metabolic fields of the child. (➤ Fig. 3.2) The child's metabolic field (in the developing abdomen) affords the most important space-occupying

process of the whole body. A Norwegian pediatrician (A. Thooris) went so far as to state that the child, until the age of three, is nothing more than "a belly"! The respiratory system requires almost four years for adapting to completed physiology. The heart depends and responds upon volume/pressure variations and positional changes of the respiratory and metabolic fields, and it will finally "sink down" from the fifth rib space to the seventh rib space at about the age of seven years.

The only action that the fully formed brain must do after completing most of its developmental phases in childhood is to descend upon the tentorium of the cerebellum and, thereby, guide the cerebellum itself to its final, adult position. In a mechanical way of thinking, one could propose that during postnatal development, the final position of the brain (the end of telencephalization/erection of the brain) requires a fully erected heart (erection of the sinus of Cuvieri, as stated by E. Blechschmidt), which itself is dependent upon the final positioning of the liver and the final gut rotation. (➤ Fig. 3.3, ➤ Fig. 3.4)

The three systems (ie, the cerebral, cardiac, and metabolic fields) are reciprocally interdependent for affording the antigravitational maturation of the baby and the continuous support of this positional integrity. Later, these same systems not only serve to express their proper physiology, but they are all interrelated for affording the upright position of the individual (erection of the body system). When the

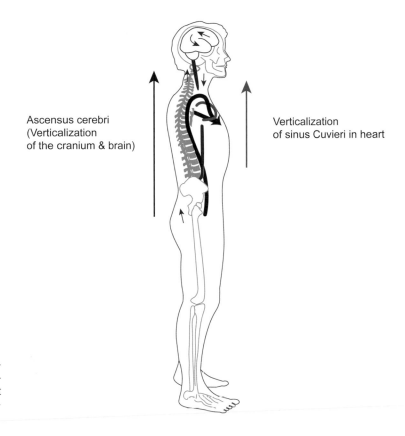

Ascensus cerebri
(Verticalization
of the cranium & brain)

Verticalization
of sinus Cuvieri in heart

Fig. 3.3 Verticalization of the body and the brain is intrinsically related to verticalization of the heart axle and its hemodynamic potential.

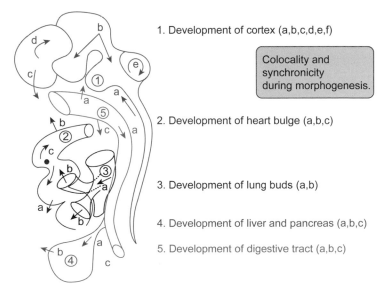

1. Development of cortex (a,b,c,d,e,f)

Colocality and
synchronicity
during morphogenesis.

2. Development of heart bulge (a,b,c)

3. Development of lung buds (a,b)

Fig. 3.4 Synchronicity between different stages of metabolic, hemodynamic, and cerebral maturation is supported by different stages of alterations in structure, form, and position.

4. Development of liver and pancreas (a,b,c)

5. Development of digestive tract (a,b,c)

erection of the body system is failing, one should consider the loss of integrity of one or all of the constituent systems (fields) in one or more of their functions. For example, in regard to the brain, a lack of erection could be expressed by an attention disorder.

Treatment and diagnosis of the child are logically dependent upon the subsequent developmental periods of the three main tissues of the body—endoderm, mesoderm, and ectoderm. In the first approach to the child, it is important for the osteopath to evaluate the integrity of the abdomen before informing the brain/skull compartment. In the second approach, it is important to evaluate the integrity of the lungs, which are partly endodermal in origin and partly mesodermal in origin.

The next step is to evaluate the freedom of the anterior and posterior parts of the mediastinum, because they indicate the relative integrity of the heart. In the final step, the osteopath can evaluate the skull/brain unit to determine if all metabolic and hemodynamic information is well integrated.

In early life, health and disease reside mostly in the belly. There, they fight on the battlefield of metabolic, endocrine, and immune equilibrium for installing a progressive order in the successive maturation processes of the homeostatic clocks of the brain. An intelligent osteopath should know about these processes before initiating treatment. For this reason, the next chapter will be centered on the topic of reciprocal information/interaction between metabolic and cerebral development during embryogenesis.

REFERENCES

[1] Heine H. Lehrbuch der Biologischen Medizin. Auflage 2. Stuttgart, Germany: Hippokrates, 1997:168.
[2] Geschwind N, Galaburda AM. Cerebral Lateralization. Cambridge, MA: Bradford Books, 1987:226–227.
[3] Lefébvre A. La fin du voyage in utero. Science et vie. 1995;190:138–141.
[4] Habib M, et al. Asymétries divergentes des aires corticales temporo-parietales: corrélations anatomo-fonctionnelles et implications évolutives et développementales. Morphologie. 1999;83(260):31–34.
[5] Magoun HI. Entrapment neuropathy in the cranium. In: Clinical Cranial Osteopathy. Meridian, ID: The Cranial Academy, 1988:186.
[6] Sutherland WG. Teachings in the Science of Osteopathy. Cambridge, MA: Rudra Press, 1990:5–6,107,218.
[7] Magoun HI. Osteopathy in the Cranial Field. Kirksville, MO: The Journal Printing Company, 1976:217–231.
[8] Brodsky L, et al. Craniofacial Anomalies: An Interdisciplinary Approach. St. Louis, MO: Mosby-Year Book, 1992:14-15,17,77,160–161.
[9] Robinson LK, et al. Vascular pathogenesis of unilateral craniofacial defects. J Pediatr. 1987;111(2):236–239.
[10] Albright AL, Byrd RP. Suture pathology in craniosynostosis. J Neurosurg. 1981;54(3):384–387.
[11] Diamond GR, et al. Variations in extraocular muscle number and structure in craniofacial dysostosis. Am J Ophthalmol. 1980;90(3):416–418.
[12] Cole P. The Respiratory Role of the Upper Airways. St. Louis, MO: Mosby-Year Book, 1993:16–19,68.
[13] Arbuckle BE. Scoliosis capitis. In: Clinical Cranial Osteopathy. Meridian, ID: The Cranial Academy, 1988:110–113.
[14] Hauser G, De Stefano GF. Epigenetic Variants of the Human Skull. Stuttgart, Germany: Schweizerbart, 1989:85–86,116,196,216.
[15] Chila A. Basic ideas about the fasciae. Presented at: Conference on the fasciae; April 8, 2001; Namur, Belgium.

The importance of osteopathic visceral techniques for the development of the young brain: a hypothesis

4.1 Introduction

We could think of the child as a young personality that steadily develops intellectual, psychological, social, and biomechanical skills [1] or we could think of the child as the result of a slowly developing biological system that sustains potential abilities in these domains. In the first case, we emphasize education. In the second case, we inform, by way of our therapeutic approach, an expansive potential of ontogenetic qualities hidden in a multipotent biological system.

As we previously mentioned, the biological system is an open system in which a multiplicity of information is integrated before the final outcome is determined. [2] Body systems are apparently organized hierarchically, but they are not strictly linked by hierarchical patterns. The interrelation between systems or functions is not only linked by neurons as a primordial source of information, but it is usually "prepared" by a substrate that potentates the final electrical and neuroendocrine pathways.

The patterning of different biological fields seems to contain the impressions of time and space related to morphogenetic processes, which are shared by synchronously developing structuring processes and functions. Although the fields don't display any linear relation with each other in an adult form (eg, a nerve relating an organ to the spinal cord or brain), they still share common mesenchymal, immune, or endocrine functions or origins. This means that the histo-anatomical hierarchy does not necessarily coincide with a hierarchy of function or subfunction in physiology. The on-and-off reaction of a motor pathway is not only determined by a reflex arc, but it is prepared by local tissue and cell modifications organizing the reaction in velocity and strength.

Organogenesis does not end at birth. Important aspects of tissue differentiation and organ space-occupying processes continue after birth. The heart descent continues until age seven, and the gut-associated lymphoid tissue increases in area and volume until age ten. Sphincter functions of the gut sometimes display immature behavior in early childhood, continuing their development through later childhood. Even the brain convolutions continue their development and differentiation in the postnatal period.

Some tissues can re-express embryological features they lost during normal development when they are obliged to function in pathological situations. The peritoneum can do so in cases of chronic kidney disease when the patient undergoes continuous ambulatory peritoneal dialysis.[1] The spleen can re-express hematopoietic function. Even the myocardium of the heart is able to reiterate embryological functions. These processes are not isolated events, but rather interrelated events guided by basic interference from biochemical and biomechanical exchanges between cells, tissues, and organs irrespective of specific progeny.

Perhaps a major part of the child's behavior that we think is dependent upon personality is actually supported by a hidden and progressive autonomic tissue adaptation to different life circumstances, ranging as widely as social and intellectual learning situations.

A few observations could help us better understand the interdependence of the developing brain and visceral sphere during childhood.

- Most illnesses during infancy are in the digestive domain and respiratory tract, indicating the

---

[1] CAPD: current ambulatory peritoneal dialysis

important role the primitive digestive tract plays in the physiological organization of homeostasis. This physiology is certainly dependent upon neurological and neurovegetative information and maturation. However, it is also, in an equivalent proportion, dependent upon tissue structuration determined by immune and metabolic stimuli.

- During embryological development, the brain matures and organizes its neural pathways from peripheral inputs provided by different neuronal growth cones that display metabolic fields with their surrounding tissue. This is a kind of "bottom-up" organization of information by the maturing tissues and organs at the periphery.
- There exists a "bilocality" of the brain. Part of the brain is centralized caudal-to-cephalad in the corticospinal tract, and part is dispersed in the tissue organizing the cardiovascular and visceral domains. Here, we can discuss "scattered clouds of peripheral brain." [3]
- The visceral domain exhibits a relative independence from the central nervous system (CNS), and it determines a major part of "the common pathway of efference" in the CNS by hormonal and molecular information.
- The visceral and neurological systems are linked by specific cell transformations and migrations realized by the neural crest cells. These cells organize a *"fourth germ layer"* that is a most important event in body organization and coordination. This basic tissue transformation occurs in the mesenchymal substrate of the growing body.
  The body homeostasis is built upon the acid-alkaline equilibrium of tissues and the hydro-electrical potentials expressed by them. When these functions are disturbed, the CNS also loses normal interference with the periphery.
- Basic chemical and physical principles of exchange in tissue determine, for a great part, the laws of generating pressure gradients, electrical field potentials, and magnetic fields of the body.
- Embryology teaches us that the differentiation of tissue and function is connected with specific genetic and time-dependent facilitation, in which the outer and inner cellular environment interplay. Biochemical and biomechanical processes use the same substrate to exchange and create basic connections between different parts of the

body during embryogenesis, and they continue to do so after birth. The mesenchymal connections and the connective tissue continue to react as a unitary fundamental substance, using the same chemical and mechanical codes as they did during embryogenesis.

- These complex exchanges are organized in both a chemical web of molecular compounds and a mechanical web called tensegrity. It is reasonable to suppose that the brain and the visceral sphere have elaborated such webs, independent of their origin.

4.2 Embryological considerations

4.2.1 Early differentiation and cell-tissue inductive systems

Cell dynamics and differentiation are dependent upon inductive processes that determine orientation and maturation of different cell lineages and germ layers. This process of induction is the basis for the creation of function and structure, and it is guided by intrinsic factors (the genome) and extrinsic factors (the chemical and mechanical environment of the cell). A specific tissue and cell differentiation will be necessary to permit chemical and mechanical interaction between cell lineages of different origin. Carlson [4] mentions that the mesoderm layer is created by the unequal growth rate between the hypoblast cell layer and the epiblastic cell layer, indicating that mechanical factors interfere with cell differentiation.

During gastrulation, some of the epiblast cells migrating through the primitive streak form the third germ layer. The mesoderm inserts itself between the epiblast and hypoblast layers. As they pass through the primitive streak, the future mesoderm cells change in morphology from epiblastic cells to "bottle cells." This mesenchymal cell lineage is a typical example of a fundamental cellular articulation between distant and distinct cell layers. Their properties of migration and transformation are based upon complex molecular events (ie, production of hyaluronic acid and fibronectin) and upon the modification of cell adhesion molecules and production of growth factors (activin, TGF-β2) (➤ Fig. 4.1). The whole process of body structuring will be dependent upon these subtle exchanges that support the ectomesenchymal, endomesenchymal, and meso-mesenchymal interference between tissues.

One of the earliest interactions that have been studied is the determining impact that the hypoblast has upon the epiblast. Mitrani and Shimoni [5], in their work on chick embryos, confirmed that by rotating the hypoblast 90° with respect to the orientation of the epiblast, the orientation of the primitive streak was altered. This type of orientation could also be possible for the human embryo.

Mesenchymal transformation could be a parallel process that organizes the molecular information in a structure dependent on the time-space relationship. The complexity of these differentiation processes seems to be stocked in a sort of memory that is not strictly genetic.

Bruce et al [6] confirm that the cell displays genetic information but adapts to environmental influences. Fibroblasts and connective tissue, in particular, display this property. This capability of adaptation of the cell is present not only throughout embryological development, but also during postnatal times. Heine [7] proposes that the diversity of sugar

polymers in the cell makes them the storage structure of choice for cellular information. Glycoproteins and proteoglycans are excellent emporiums in which chemical and mechanical inputs can be linked. The fibroblast, which originates in the early embryological mesenchymal tissue, seems to be the trigger mechanism mediating structural and functional transformations (➤ Fig. 4.2).

Growth factors [8, 9] are continuously interfering with tissue adaptations, regeneration, and repair in prenatal and postnatal stages, as well as in adulthood. Tissue has the capability to integrate a part of the "ontogenetic momentum" in its final functional structure. Hinrischen [10] and other authors [11] confirm that the pericardium integrates the mechanical evolutions of the heart rotations during embryological development, in the orientation of its collagen and elastin fibrils.

We may suggest that a large part of these interactions continue to exist in postnatal life, and they possibly contribute to continuous adaptations in changing physiological circumstances.

One conclusion we may propose is that the basic principle of tissue interaction and transformation is an early cell differentiation process that is used to induce most of the structuring events in tissue and viscera. These processes are essentially based upon ectomesenchymal and epithelio-mesenchymal

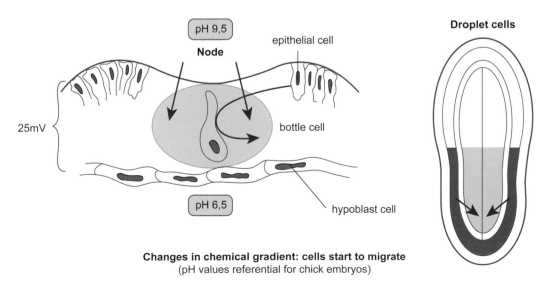

Changes in chemical gradient: cells start to migrate
(pH values referential for chick embryos)

Fig. 4.1 Epithelial to mesenchymal transformation at the level of the node and migration of bottle cells—one of the primordial features for mesenchymal patterning of the embryonic landscape

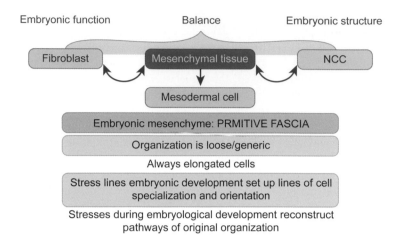

Fig. **4.2** The mesenchymal cell/tissue represents the balance between fibroblast activity and early NCC activity. This balance could play a role in further adaptations and reaction patterns in fully differentiated tissue.

inductive processes. As Carlson states [12], these inductions sustain the metabolic and mechanical actions of tissues and organs.

A second possible conclusion is that the hypoblast and early endoderm cells, as well as the primitive gut, display inductive possibilities on the early neural tube to direct and to intensify the growth and orientation of this tube. There is a striking demonstration of the stimulating powers of the gut. Pieces of gut wall (ie, mesoderm) transplanted along the neural tube cause a great expansion of the region of the neural tube closest to the graft. There are additional factors in the gut wall that stimulate the mitosis of the neural crest cells migrating in that area.

4.2.2 Hierarchy in body systems and function

A second striking point in tissue differentiation is that this tissue organization needs metabolic support to develop its specialized functions. Every specialization of tissue is, in fact, a metabolic field in which the laws of cellular and tissue exchange are primordial. Part of the dynamic properties of cells can be understood by studying the principles of biodynamic, biokinetic mechanisms that build structure, form, and spaces in the developing body, as suggested by Blechschmidt and Gasser. [13] These principles state that every structure, form, and function is built on three dynamic properties of cells and tissue:

- electrophysiological exchange
- nourishing currents (transmembranous electrical potential, thermal gradient, space)
- degradation of currents (inducing cell apoptosis).

It can be further stated that the molecular and electrophysiological equilibrium determine exchange of metabolites and the tonality (tension, elasticity, and mobility) of tissue. The polarization of the body prepares it for the possibility of exchange (metabolism), coaptation (strength), and mobility (movement).

The growth of the brain makes it an intensive expanding metabolic field that causes the blood circulation to increase. It is the enlargement of the heart that permits the increased metabolic support to the brain. If there were not an increased metabolic need from the brain, the liver would not expand and begin its early metabolic activity (ie, glycogenesis and hematopoiesis).

The brain is largely dependent upon the metabolic activity and circulatory increase throughout the whole body. Blechschmidt and Gasser refer to these phases of tissue maturation and specification as "hepatization," "cardialization," and "cerebralization." [13] These landmarks of tissue interdependence are not only important to establish organ function but also to direct the spatial organization of the body plan (➤ Fig. 4.3).

The expanding liver appears to function as a filter for blood before it courses to the heart. The increase in the liver circumference causes the diaphragm to flatten. which is important for the descent of the viscera and the resulting origin of the nasal and bronchopulmonary portion of the pulmonary tract.

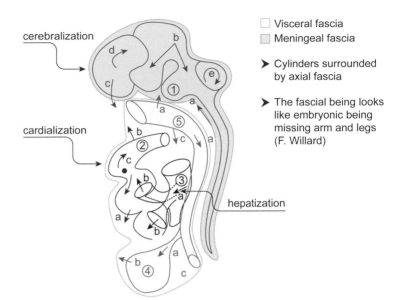

cerebralization

cardialization

hepatization

☐ Visceral fascia
▨ Meningeal fascia

➤ Cylinders surrounded by axial fascia

➤ The fascial being looks like embryonic being missing arm and legs (F. Willard)

Fig. 4.3 The primitive fasciae (splanchnopleura and dural membranes) play an intrinsic role in guiding the different compartments of the body into different plans of interference. By this means, each compartment functions as a field that can interfere with other fields.

These different biodynamic processes organize progressively separated but interrelated fascial compartments, which were defined by F. Willard[2] as being the internal fasciae.

These fasciae participate at the global "Gestaltung" of the visceral body that is linked to the CNS. Here also the memory of the brain is based upon biodynamical principles that built up the architectural complexity of the body plan.

This creates another important point that outlines the intimate relationship between brain development and visceral organization. The fact that both areas display opposite and interrelated movements to construct their final anatomical emplacement makes them functionally and anatomically related by the organization of their fascial compartments. Not only are they organized reciprocally, but the intrinsic patterning in one fascial compartment means that each space-occupying process interferes with an analogue process in the other compartment. For example, part of the looping of the heart and its septation can be linked to processes at brain level that organize the brain flexures or the movement of brain compaction (➤ Fig. 4.4). [14]

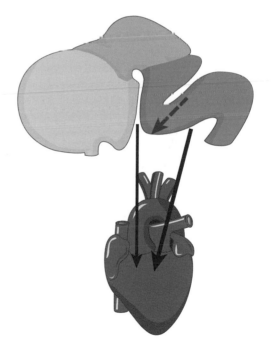

Fig. 4.4 Mechanical interference at a distance between a cerebral flexure and heart orientation

To better understand the importance of these synchronous biodynamical interferences, we can consider some of the more classical landmarks of these processes in reference to the anatomy of the adult

[2] Willard F. Conference on fasciae; 2012; Brussels, Belgium.

body. This consideration should make the reader aware of the fact that anatomy is not only linear but space- and time-related.

Caudal movement of the viscera is referred to as a "descent primarily relative to the brain." A well-known manifestation of visceral descent is the innervation of the diaphragm by the phrenic nerve, which arises from the spinal cord segment C4. In a similar manner, the developmental movement of the entire neural tube is conceived as ascending (ie, cranial movement of the neural tube relative to the intestine.) A typical example of ascent is the progressive formation of the cauda equina from the roots of lumbar and sacral spinal nerves, which course vertically in the vertebral canal. Another example is the progressive protrusion of the embryonic forehead of the upper neural tube. [13]

Intrinsic structural transformation of the brain may be supported by mechanical events necessary for cell differentiation and migration, as suggested by E.N. Emmanouil-Nikoloussi, et al: [15] *"Neural tube closure in the cervical area (closure 1) begins at the location where the bend in the embryo exists, which tends to bring the two folds of the neural crest together. This fact suggests, according to Jacobson and Tam (1982), that this bend may mechanically assist the closure in this cervical region. There is a second closure, (closure 2), which overlies the bend, the cranial flexure. The direction of this flexure probably tends to spread the neural folds apart, and is expected to have an impediment to closure. Each major region of the forming neural tube may request unique combination of mechanisms to provide the force for elevation of the neural folds".*

The development of the different fascial structures enveloping the spinal cord seems to be essential for permitting this ascent of the neural tube against the other structures of the embryonic body. Dural, pial, and arachnoidal sleeves produce a pressure gradient, constituted by progressive arachnoidal liquor secretion, that permits this ascent (➤ Fig. 4.5). [16]

We could suggest that every change in structure and function is accompanied by:
- metabolic exchange between different compartments,
- displacement of differentiating forms in space,
- altering functions dependent upon the environmental influence of the specific space occupied by a pre-organ form.

The best example is the kidney, which differentiates under different pre-forms (ie, fractals) dependent upon particular anatomical places. The pronephros, mesonephros, and metanephros each occupy a specific topography and display a specific function. The pronephros occupies the embryonic neck region, serving only to induce the formation of pronephric ducts, which grow to the cloaca. They stimulate the intermediate mesoderm, leading to the formation of

Neural Crest

Nervous System

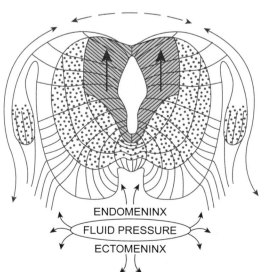

Fig. 4.5 The mechanical contact and pressure traction events between ectomeninx and endomeninx induce the production of a "fluid cushion" that permits gliding and positioning of the spinal cord.

mesonephric ducts and the mesonephron, which produces a kind of pro-urine. The mesonephros disappears by compression of the expanding liver.

The metanephros represents the final articulation between the metanephrogenic blastema and the ureteric bud. It is composed of three mesodermal pieces of information: the ureteric bud, the blastemal mesenchym, and the ingrowing vascular endothelial cells. The produced urine, serving as a pressure gradient in the urethra, guarantees its ascent in the retroperitoneal space. Growth factors (NGF, EGF) serve as attracting substances to induce migration of the kidney into the neighborhood of the descending diaphragm.

However, the most important event could be the reintegration of the so-called "physiological hernia" of the primitive gut into the abdomen, which imposes a rotational force of 270° to the peritoneal sac in a counterclockwise direction.

Here again, we may suggest that mechanical and molecular events in different parts of the body synchronize the construction plan of neighboring structures and functions. By the tenth week, the abdominal cavity has enlarged sufficiently to accommodate the intestinal tract. The intestinal loops start to move through the intestinal ring and into the abdominal cavity, integrating the coils the gut made outside the embryonic body. During these coiling, herniations, and return movements, the intestines are suspended from the dorsal body wall by mesentery. As the intestines assume their definitive positions within the body cavity, the mesentery follows and integrates part of the coils in its radix (motion and tension), but with its center of insertion at the dorsal body wall.

Parts of the mesentery associated with the duodenum and colon (mesoduodenum and mesocolon) fuse with the peritoneal lining of the dorsal body wall [12], creating a valvelike organization around the different branching arteries of the aorta. The superior and inferior mesenteric arteries are constricted by these valvelike insertions of the primitive mesentery around their origin.

One can imagine that when there is destabilization of the peritoneal content (eg, by ptosis), these valves become more or less tensed and exert a resistive force upon the systolic pulsations of the heart. This is the process that A.T. Still described in his story about the

goat and the bolder. To summarize this story: When the heart, during its systolic movement, expulses the blood to the periphery of the body and the organs, it must rely upon a relaxed passage of the aorta through the diaphragm's aortic opening. When there is tension at this opening, the blood rebounds within the aortic bed and needs to find another way out (such as to the spleen or inside the mediastinal or cranio/cervical vascular beds). In that case, the blood behaves like a goat bouncing its head against a boulder. This same principle can be applied to other vascular restrictions or constrictions.

The insertion of the primitive mesentery not only is concentrated upon vascular branches, but it also interacts with other fasciae, which develop within the retroperitoneal space of the kidneys. Fusion between the fascia of Toldt and the perirenal fasciae of Gerota apparently constitutes the frame of the anatomical articulation between the colon and the kidney.

A few conclusions may be suggested:

- Structure and function display a fractal-like evolution in preparation for definitive function and spatial emplacement.
- Spatial organization of the embryonic body is governed by two main actors—the neural tube and the primitive gut—and correlated by ever-adapting mesenchyme proliferation.
- Both actors display an ascending-versus-descending movement that is coordinated at the same time with a 270° counterclockwise rotation of the gut, which seems to stabilize the retroperitoneal and intraperitoneal spaces reciprocally.
- The final ascent and protrusion of the forebrain is blocked by development of the organs (mainly the heart) and their fascial components, when the process of intestinal looping and fixations also comes to an end.
- We can suggest that some of the structuring of the brain and viscera continues after birth:
  - brain circumvolutions continue to increase in number
  - epithelial-mesenchymal induction continues
  - descent of viscera continues.

These suggestions indicate that the structure-function relationship probably continues to use, at least partly, the same laws of genesis found in the embryonic and fetal period. Inversely, there exists increasing agreement about the fact that, under certain circumstances, specialized tissues (eg, heart, kidney) can recapitulate events that occur in the normal course of embryogenesis. [5, 17] *"Biomechanical features never occur beside chemical features, but they always implicate the latter."* [13] (p.XIV)

4.2.3 Maturation and postnatal development

Self-evidently, most of the molecular interactions, epithelial-mesenchymal induction events, and even mechanical displacements continue after birth. Hinrischen [7] states, *„Offenbar setzt sich ganz allgemein der Descensus der Eingeweide bis in das Greisenalter fort, wie klinische Berichte über die Altersptosis der inneren Organe lehren."* (English translation: Apparently the descensus viscerum continues until old age, as clinical information on ptosis of viscera suggests.) This also offers a logical reason to believe that mechanical compartments continue to interfere, to some extent, with each other at the moment that the osseous and fascial envelopes become more rigid.

Perhaps the most striking point in perinatal and postnatal evolution is that there are apparently two main structures that differentiate in this crucial period. Certainly, the brain is subjected to profound reorganization of established neural pathways, in which cellular apoptosis plays an important organizational role. This reorganization seems to continue until puberty [18], underlining the importance of cranial techniques during this period.

Another important point is the enormous increase in mass of the lymphoid tissue and the 200% increase of immune system maturation until the age of ten. This fact indicates that the immune system is probably the most important structure that makes survival and integration of exogenous stimuli (antigenic stimuli) possible for the young body. The largest part of this process is related to the glands and structures associated with the development of the endoderm layer.

The thymus plays a key role in the maturation of T-lymphocytes and B-lymphocytes. It acts as an important dispatching center to the spleen and the peripheral lymph organs associated with the gut—the gut-associated lymphoid tissue (GALT). Serial

studies in animals have shown that Peyer's patches in early stages are populated chiefly by thymus-derived T-cells. Activated cells in Peyer's patches seem to migrate throughout the body, selectively populating the lamina propria of the intestinal mucosa, where they form the extensive plasma cell population. They also migrate to the bronchial and genitourinary tracts and to the mammary, salivary, and lachrymal glands. Bronchial mucosal lymphoblasts apparently migrate reciprocally to the intestinal mucosa. These migrations have been demonstrated for B-cells, and it is believed that T-cells behave similarly. [19]

We can note that the extensive development of the immune system covers an area extending from the epithelium of the middle ear and throat to the whole surface of the gut and lungs, in addition to the genitourinary tract and lachrymal glands. The thymus attains its maximum mass at sexual maturity (puberty). After puberty, there is a striking involution in the size of the thymus, so that a person of 40 to 50 years retains only 5% to 10% of the gland's cellular mass.

We can state that the development of the immune system expresses a similar, if not a more important, degree of activity and transformation as the developing brain until puberty. It certainly is as important as the brain for the survival of the individual as a result of its capacity to integrate exogenous antigenic stimuli. The immune system could be conceived of as a mobile peripheral brain, or a sixth sense, that informs the body and brain by the two pathways of cellular and humoral defense mechanisms.

It is accepted that the immune system and the neuro-endocrine system are linked to each other by common receptors and ligands. [20] Sari et al [21] confirm that the interleukins secreted by the T-lymphocytes, especially IL-1 and IL-2, are found at the hypothalamic and hypocampic levels, representing a manner of molecular dialogue between the immune system and the brain. The reticulo-endothelial system that surrounds and structures the thymus seems capable of interference by its own secretions with pituitary hormones and other neuropeptides, including gonadotropic hormone (GH), prolactin, adrenocorticotropic hormone (ACTH), thyroid stimulating hormone (TSH), somatostatin (SOM), follicle stimulating hormone (FSH), and luteinizing hormone (LH). [22]

All this underlines the magnitude of influence that the immune system may exert on the developing brain, as well as how the visceral system—by the way of GALT (gut-associated lymphoid tissue) and BALT (bronchus-associated lymphoid tissue)— may interfere with normal processes in the brain of the youngster. The cytokines secreted during inflammatory or infectious episodes may alter the local metabolic and mechanical physiology of the intestine, and they might also interfere with cytokine release at other places of the body (eg, the brain) by humoral passageways.

A provisional conclusion we might suggest is that during early infancy, there are two major systems competing with each other to install a certain hegemony, each of them belonging to a different developmental origin—the brain as a specialized ectoderm tissue and the immune system as a specialization of the endoderm and mesoderm germ layers. Because of their parallel development and search for dialoguing (ie, interaction, interference, exchange), it is not impossible that perturbations in one field are transmitted to the other field by way of molecular (cytokine), neurohormonal, and direct neural pathways (ie, sympathetic and parasympathetic connections between the neurovegetative system and the singular lymphocytes or the lymph-organs, thymus, spleen, and GALT).

Another assessment concerns the role that the reticulo-endothelial system (RES) plays in structuring and fixing the major lymph-organs. We may propose a simultaneous defensive and mechanical role for this structure. Its role can be compared to the function of the fundamental substance as described by Pischinger.[2] It could integrate and dispatch mechanical and molecular inputs at the same time. This means that defensive impulses and mechanical impulses (motility and mobility of the viscera) are probably vectored largely over the same pathway to the brain and vice versa.

The immune system and the RES, which contains the major information of the extracellular matrix, represent two important feedback systems to the CNS. By this means, they condition much of the neuro-endocrine, autonomous, and neurocognitive interferences of the brain with the inner body and the outer environmental stimuli. In a certain sense, one could state that what is perceived in the outer world is preconditioned by the internal state of the immune system and the vegetative state of the body.

4.3 Pathological patterns in postnatal development of the gastrointestinal tract: a time schedule and its possible usefulness in interpreting normal physiology

By studying the time of appearance of certain pathologies in pediatrics, one can remark that there exist critical periods in which some affections of the gut are more pronounced. [23]

- Pyloric stenosis usually appears between the 15th and 40th day after a symptom-free period of almost two weeks. The causes are related to an absence of intramural ganglia and, according to some authors, a delay in maturation of certain nuclei of the vagal nerve. We know that the mesodermal layer of the intestine exerts a trophic and attractant force upon migrating neural crest cells. However, few studies have been made of how a sphincter is generated. From a biodynamic viewpoint [24] it could be acceptable that the multitude of rotations of the primitive gut play an important role in concentrating mesoderm in specific places of strain, torsion, and compression of this structuring layer. It could also be conceivable that the whole process of spatial organization is not finished at birth but continues for a short time after. That could explain the "late" appearance of this stenosis. The main problem could be a mechanical impact on that specific place by a not fully organized peritoneal sac. Another possibility could be that the vagal area at the brainstem site was impacted by some mechanical aggression during parturition.
- Ileocecal, ileocolic, and ileo-ileac impacting constitute the greatest abdominal urgency in infants between the fourth and ninth month, and it is the most frequent cause of intestinal occlusion during that period of life. Although the cause is not well known, the impacting is sometimes preceded

by an infectious episode of the rhino pharynx or enteric domain. It is clear that a mechanical event could be induced by disturbance of intramural and previsceral reflexes that are activated by infectious or toxic pathogens. Those pathogens interfere with the motor patterns present in the ileum and proximal colon.

- Appendicitis rarely appears before the age of three. Afterwards, it commonly appears as an expression of an altered state of the intestine due to local or more generalized inflammatory processes of the gut. The exact cause is not clearly described, but the symptoms often raise doubts regarding whether the condition is real appendicitis or a lymphadenitis of the mesentery. Definitive diagnosis is often made during surgery.
- At a later age (8–12 years), appendicitis may be accompanied or caused by other factors contributing to sexual maturation (gonad/appendix), indicating a hormonal interference.

Three types of aggression could cause this inflammatory process—hyperstimulation of the concentrated GALT at that level (lymphadenitis mesenterica), irritation by the enterohepatic cycle (secondary bile salt absorption), or hormonal, mechanical, and positional unbalance of the appendix (retrocaecal). Similar time schedules could probably be found in the cardiac or pulmonary domains (eg, time limits to operate Fallot's tetralogy, coarctation of the aorta, and appearance of asthma versus eczema).

Some conclusions are suggested concerning the pathology of the gastrointestinal tract in the neonate and infant:

- Most of the pathology previously mentioned is the result of synergy between two types of tissue interfering with each other—the immune system of the gut (mucosa-lamina propria) and the motor system (muscularis mucosa, circular, and longitudinal muscle layers). They interact via chemosensitive and mechanosensitive intramural pathways determining the intramural reflexes. The immune system of the gut is also influenced by sympathetic input, which further influences the motor patterns of the gut. Over-reactivity of the immune system apparently interferes with normal motor patterns of the gut.
- Local rhinopharyngeal or respiratory infectious attacks can elicit or facilitate inflammatory episodes

in the gut, indicating that the superficial layers of the gut epithelium function as a whole and are probably coordinated by the disseminated GALT. This implies that the diseases of the throat or middle ear (otitis media) could be generated locally or at a distance by metabolic or mechanical disturbances of the gut and vice versa.

- The peritoneum could be an important mediator in creating local spasm and inhibition of mobility and motility, as seen in the cases of volvulus and appendicitis.
- The normal development of the mesodermal layer of the gut is an important attractant for migrating neural crest cells, which could partly explain the appearance of certain pathologies, such as pyloric stenosis and Hirschsprung's disease. However, we notice that the peritoneum plays an important role in the spatial organization of the gut, and that malrotation or defective maturation of this tissue could determine part of these pathologies.
- Certain pathologies are typical for a lifetime, which underscores that the chronology and topography of syndromes are related to immaturity of some organizing tissues (ie, peritoneum and lymphoid tissue) in their spatial and functional development. Pathology can be linked to specific pathogens, but, at the same time, it could be organized by deficient rotation or position of the immature peritoneal or pleural-cardiac cavities.

4.4 Interference between the brain and the visceral sphere

Korr [25] states that the sympathetic nervous system interconnects the visceral physiology with the brain. This indicates a certain independence between both functions, which have to rely for a large part upon the peripheral sympathetic system to interfere.

The functions of the intramural plexuses of Auerbach and Meissner are so complex that they are described as the "peripheral brain." Furthermore, it is true that central controls are not strictly hierarchical, but rather arranged as an interactive system, responsive to somatic as well as visceral afferents.

Information from several levels may influence the final efferent command. It is well established that go and no-go decisions are made throughout widely ramified centers of autonomic pathways in response to signals from ascending as well as from descending connections at various levels of the neuraxis, including the spinal cord, medulla, hypothalamus, thalamus, cerebellar and limbic pathways, and frontal lobes. [26]

Subtle exchanges between the chemical and mechanical compartments of the gut create a vast array of intramural, previsceral, prevertebral, and medullar reflexes in which the interplay between chemical and mechanical coding of mucosa, submucosa, and muscle layers assumes a determining role. Even mechanoreceptors in the peritoneum, either under the serosa of the viscus near the mesenteric connections or in the mesentery and omentum, are generally associated with the splanchnic nerves. These receptors respond to distortion of the viscera and are considered to be involved in mediating visceral pain, though from the receptor sensitivities they may also play a role in reflex regulation of GI function. [27]

The splanchnic nerves and the vagal afference seem only to underline the importance of the informing ability upon the brain. The meaning is that a great part of this final efferent command of the brain is ultimately determined by visceral "sensations," which are implicated in behavioral changes, such as satiety, nausea, and vomiting.

The gut and the peritoneum display the capability of secreting a wide array of molecular compounds, ranging from hormones and prostaglandins to cytokines, many of which interfere with the physiology of the brain. As Rehfeld states, *"Gastrointestinal hormones should be viewed not only as local hormones of interest for digestive physiologists and clinical gastroenterologists. It is not surprising that classic gut hormones today are studied not only in physiology, pharmacology, biochemistry, and cell biology, but also by psychologists, psychiatrists, zoologists, molecular oncologists, diabetologists, and others. It is possible and even likely that most regulatory peptides (hormones, neurotransmitters, growth hormones, cytokines) at least at some stage in the phylogenetic or ontogenetic development are expressed in the gut."* [28]

Vasoactive intestinal peptide (VIP) was studied for its effect upon cerebral vascularization and the enhancement of choroid plexus blood flow. It is reasonable to believe that the gut translates some of its metabolic of mechanical activity by altering local and distant blood circulation. [29, 30] Even growth hormones display a determining role in generating pathological processes that find their roots in early development of function and structure. There exists a direct relationship between growth and differentiation processes in early development and pathological processes in the adult. Many growth factors (IGF, FGF, TGF-β) are multifunctional regulatory molecules exerting diverse biological effects upon the identity of the target cells with which they interact. [5]

The peritoneum displays an enormous role in this complex physiology. Through its ability to react upon mechanical stimuli, such as friction between opposite layers of its mesothelial lining and mechanical compression or distention, it produces a vast array of prostaglandins, which exert cytoprotective activity. "Mechanical stimulation is known to increase the release of arachidonic acid, which could lead to an increased formation of metabolites with vasodilating, permeability increasing, and mucus-generating activity. An increased release of arachidonic acid could be the result of the continuous friction between the opposite layers of the mesothelium," [31]

There is also evidence of the gut and peritoneum trying to resolve their problems independently of other systems. It is at the level of the peritoneum that we can best notice how interdependently the local enteric nervous system (ENS) interferes with stimuli of metabolic or immune order. The cells of the immune system and the mediators they synthesize—particularly the cytokines and other mediators of inflammation, the leukotriens, prostaglandins, and histamine—all participate actively in the development of pathology in the nervous system, endocrine system, and smooth muscle physiology. Recent studies prove that, conversely, the smooth muscle and the ENS also influence the immune system. The activity of the intestinal motricity during colitis, for example, seems to be the result of interrelations between the immune system, ENS, and smooth muscle. [32]

Another important fact is that during early stages of development of the gastrointestinal tract (approximately the fourth to eighth week), an informative cell population (neural crest cells) descends to the previsceral and/or intramural ganglia. There, the NCC's orchestrate the major part of visceral and previsceral reflex activity. One can see that two major domains exist in the previsceral and intramural compartments of the gut that display a more or less dominant role depending upon their location of early colonization. The parasympathetic system seems more dominant at the level of the stomach and sigmoid complex. The sympathetic system seems more dominant at the level of the intestinal tract and ileocecal junction.

The neural crest cells function at that moment as early messengers of molecular orders integrated in the regionalization of the anterior, middle, and posterior intestinal portals. In a certain way, they transmit early space/time scales shared between the developing CNS and the gut ENS (➤ Fig. 4.6).

Conclusions we may suggest include the following:
- The gut and the peritoneum possess their proper nervous system, the ENS, which is capable of integrating different types of stimuli in local reflex mechanisms and through adaptations in metabolic, defensive, and motor tonus.

- The molecular and hormonal arsenal secreted by the gut and peritoneum is similar to the circulating and local molecular and hormonal substances we find in the brain, indicating a certain form of communication that extends across the barriers of their specific functions.
- Both systems interfere with each other by a common "go between": the sympathetic nervous system seems interposed between the CNS and the ENS.
- The CNS is in almost direct anatomical contact with extensions of the gut system. The mucosa of the gut and the lymph organs extend as far as the middle ear, sometimes even into the mastoid cells. The same can be said about the rhinopharynx, which extends into the base of the skull, including into the parotid space (n. VII), carotid space (nn. IX, X), and masticator space (n. V). [33]

Finally, we could observe that the brain is subjected to information of the visceral system by three ways of signaling:
- the nervous common pathway of signaling
- the immune system linked codes: prostaglandins, cytokines, leukotriens

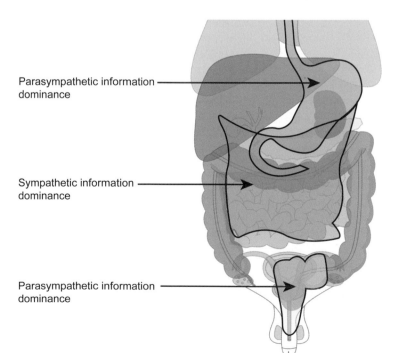

Parasympathetic information dominance

Sympathetic information dominance

Parasympathetic information dominance

Fig. 4.6 The enteric nervous system of the gut represents a "second brain" in the body. The sympathetic information (blue) is centered by parasympathetic domains (yellow).

- anatomical contact dependent upon the integrity of the internal limiting fascia—for example, the meninges and the fascia that limit the spaces of the visceral compartments of the neck and thoracic-abdominal spaces.

4.5 Osteopathic considerations

The only way for the osteopath to interfere with a body system—whether immune, digestive, cardiopulmonary, or cranial—is to interfere with the system's anatomical parts, which translate some of their function to the palpating hand. There is a growing amount of evidence that a single structure may express different forms of activity to fulfill a particular function. The best example may be that of the peritoneal mesothelium, which expresses activities for secreting substances (prostaglandins), draining and production of lymph, repair of tissue, defense of tissue against infectious attacks, integration of defensive neural signals, and coordinating stability and mobility of vascular beds and of the organs themselves.

Most of these enumerated functions are dependent upon one particular property of the mesothelium, namely friction. [34] The peritoneum needs freedom of its tissue to display friction moments that generate all of its functions. This means that the peritoneum is particularly sensitive to mechanical distortion and fixation, which impedes its function.

Thus, the peritoneum should be considered as an organ, rather than a simple envelope, that is more or less distorted by intestinal looping and fixations at the back of the thoracic-abdominal cavity. By its physiological integrity, it plays a major role in integrating vascular, neuroendocrine, and autonomous reflexes and, in most cases, it is able to resolve inflammatory and traumatic events very locally and very rapidly (within two days) through tissue repair and molecular interference with its environment (fibrosis).

The peritoneum presents as a tissue that can integrate local information. It serves as a database for past events through subtle changes in its chemical-electrical reaction patterns, which are organized by molecular stimuli (cytokines) or mechanical

exchange (friction, pressure). By its intimate relationship with the CNS, it shares part of the basic information of our consciousness that is triggered by visceroception, and it forms the basis for our cognitive and emotional processing through its sense of the physiological condition of the body (interoception).

We suppose that this was one of the reasons that W.G. Sutherland advised his students to have a keen and soft access to the peritoneum, and to not be too aggressive or invasive with their palpatory techniques for this tissue.

The first automatism an osteopath displays when he or she has to treat a baby or child is to touch the head (cranium) of the youngster, as if all the magic of life was hidden behind this chondroid bowl. The peritoneum is a tissue that is much more superficial and just as dynamic as the developing brain and nerves. Its importance can be highlighted by the following points:

- It guarantees stability, exchange, and mobility of the gut and abdomen.
- It creates pressure gradients that permit exchange between thoracic and intracranial pressure.
- It is sensitive to compression and stretch, and it reacts as a fundamental substance (ECM).
- As the brain in the cranium, it has not found its definite position in the belly. It continues to rotate and to install anatomical relationships between the gut and its environment, especially during the first three years of life.

Every osteopath should be capable of guaranteeing the vitality and orientation of this tissue by sustaining its search for final stability, by freeing early adhesions or fixations, and by repeating effective maneuvers as frequently as needed. However, one could ask oneself what an osteopath is really doing when manipulating a cranium.

- Is the osteopath manipulating the bones by moving them, or is he or she simply molding chondroid bones through pressure?
- Is the osteopath interfering with the brain directly by the intermediate of the cranium or by the reciprocal tension membranes?
- Is the osteopath interfering with the periphery through pure neurological pathways?
- Could it also be possible that the osteopath is interfering with a dynamic field that—in its own way and dependent upon its own prevalence—

reacts upon a mechanical stimulus by modifying the parameters necessary to guarantee homeostasis related to its function?

This last point would mean that a neurological field guarantees some parameters of homeostasis, as does the metabolic field. Some adaptations are specific to the particular function (eg, neurological or metabolic impulses), and others are more dependent upon the tissue surrounding the dynamic field (eg, the meninges or the peritoneum). It is conceivable that a mechanical impulse activates a specialized reaction and, at the same time, facilitates specific tissue adaptations that organize and connect different dynamical fields. In this way, a cranial technique could influence the neurological field while simultaneously interfering with a metabolic field using two types of signaling.

A manipulation cannot induce a specific quantity of adrenaline by acting upon a stellate ganglion. Neither can it control the amount of molecular compounds released during a visceral technique on the stomach. The only expectation that is reasonable is that a manipulation facilitates the interaction between an organizing and a connecting tissue, which possesses its own way of influencing the underlying function—in this case, the stellate ganglion or the stomach.

As we previously studied in the embryological considerations, the mesenchymal tissue can be conceived of as the result of mechanical interactions between two main tissues—the ectoderm and the endoderm. Independently of whether it deals with a structure or a specific form or function, this transformation of tissue continues to be functional throughout life. This fact suggests that it is probably possible to stimulate tissue adaptations throughout life, as studies done on connective tissue show us. [4, 18]

We could conceive of the fibroblast as a local manufacturer of transformations and the mastocyte as a messenger capable of informing the brain without implicating neural pathways. [35] What is called "specialized tissue"—such as the tissue of the brain, gut, and muscles—is actually the executor of a cellular code that facilitates or inhibits adaptive function to a changing environment. The physical and chemical laws that organize physiology also determine, for a great deal, the capability and the quality of our cognitive functions.

The physical laws integrated into osteopathic philosophy and medicine are probably simpler than most theories elaborated until now. It could be that the act of compressing a system (ie, a specialized tissue organization) is sufficient to elicit a broad array of integrated reaction patterns that express themselves in neurological circuits, chemical patterns, or even mechanical patterns that are slightly moderated in frequency, force, or time of execution of specific tasks.

Manipulating an abdomen is, in fact, nothing else than the addition of pressure to a specific anatomical level, accompanied by a sharp but gentle contact facilitating the parameters of motion, depth, and direction of the manipulating hand. When one compresses the abdomen, one is increasing the abdominal pressure by the physical law of adding energy and resistance to expansion. This might be sufficient to not only increase pressure but also to favor a specific tissue reaction that facilitates the adaptation capability of the abdomen by well-established reaction pathways. The release of hormones and neural facilitation could be the consequence of facilitating reaction patterns at the tissue level. The best example is the mesothelial cell of the peritoneum, which requires friction, a mechanical impulse, to free prostaglandins and to favor most of its defense and metabolic activities.

Applying these parameters of treatment in the pediatric field is especially interesting, because it might be that one is not only treating a specific anatomical field, but also giving additional impulses that permit maturation, elaboration, or reinforcement of new pathways. It could be that neurological, immune, or endocrine reaction patterns are strengthened by the laws of tensegrity, through increasing plasticity of the body systems.[3] The main importance of osteopathic techniques in the pediatric field is that the application of compressive techniques could stimulate tissue maturation when executed with respect to biological and biomechanical parameters of development.

---

[3] Compression or stretch exerts an activating impulse upon the elastic system of the body by, for example, transformation of collagen type I or II into type IV.

Another important point is that the body systems (eg, cranial, cardiovascular, metabolic fields) are not strictly organized in a hierarchical manner. They interfere by biophysical laws of pressure gradients and electrical potentials that can dominate the hierarchy of the brain upon the other systems. [36] Abdominal pressure, for example, influences cranial pressure and can alter the neurological integrity of the brain.

Tissue integrity is primarily dependent upon local metabolic exchange (osmotic, oncotical, hydroelectric values; electrochemical exchanges) before interfering with more specialized areas of the body. Local activity is an expression of a trial to resolve physiological needs on the spot. Only thereafter could more generalized reaction patterns organize.

Apparently, a reiteration of embryological evolutionary patterns, in which local activity and cell specification serve as trophic factors, integrates an increasingly centralized way of organization. The brain is "fed" by peripheral stimuli, which permits it to mature and to develop more complex reaction patterns. This process can be viewed as a "bottom-up" flow of information that progressively increases the potential of the brain to integrate information and to develop patterns of interference that function, in turn, in a "top-down" manner. It amounts to an effective way of expressing reactivity upon the inner and outer environment of the individual. By integrating increasingly more reactive patterns, the brain adds microtimes of consciousness to the basic program of its genetic and epigenetic parameters.

L. Vandervert [37] defines this process as a space-time neuromatrix, in which complex patterns of integration are increasingly stacked into the brain structure and in the little "box" called the "skull." This process has been studied during phylogenetic development of the different phyla: *"The common basic design of brains and nervous systems across phyla illustrates that the evolution of algorithms that deal with space and time contingencies, for example, those of the brain's hippocampus, the evolutionary floor of the cerebral cortex extends back in time over hundreds of millions of years. … the human brain can be viewed as carrying in it a triune paleontology of consciousness that involves that of reptiles, prehominid mammals, and humans."*

Interaction between the main systems of the body is not necessarily dependent upon structural continuity or upon hierarchical structuration. For example, the cardiovascular system is influenced by:

- hydrostatic forces and peripheral vascular resistance
- hormones secreted from different sources (eg, thyroid, adrenal)
- autonomic nerve system
- bulbar impulses, themselves influenced by respiratory oscillatory neurons reacting upon H+ concentration in the CSF
- hemoglobin-oxygen load in circulating red blood cells, influencing simultaneously the respiratory system and neural autonomous pathways.

Information can use different biological pathways, including neurological, endocrine, and circulatory, as well as different physical laws, including hydrostatic pressure and hydroelectrical fields. The osteopath should keep these different passageways in mind as possible action fields that react in a "source-and-pit" pattern, which omits the strict hierarchical and linear organization of the body.

REFERENCES
[1] De Ajuriaguerra J. Manuel de Psychiatrie de l'enfant. France: Masson, 1973:1–144.
[2] Pischinger A. Das System der Grundregulation. 7 Auflage. Heidelberg, Germany: Haug Verlag, 1985.
[3] Grundy D, Read NW. Clinical Gastroenterology. Kent, United Kingdom: Baillière-Tindal, 1988.
[4] Carlson M.B. Human Embryology and Developmental Biology. St Louis, MO: Mosby-Year Book, 1994:51–64.
[5] Mitrani E, Shimoni Y. Induction by soluble factors of organized axial structures in chick epiblasts. Science. 1990;247(4946):1092–1094.
[6] Bruce A, et al. Biologie moléculaire de la cellule. 3rd ed. Paris, France: Flammarion Medecine-Sciences, 1994:34, 1140–1142.
[7] Heine H. Lehrbuch der biologischen Medizin. Stuttgart, Germany: Hippokrates Verlag, 1997:33,41.
[8] Heath JK, Smith AG. Growth factors in embryogenesis. Br Med Bull. 1989;45(2):319–336.
[9] Hammerman MR, et al. Role of growth factors in regulation of renal growth. Annu Rev Physiol. 1993;55:305–321.
[10] Hinrichsen KV. Human Embryologie. Heidelberg, Germany: Springer Verlag, 1990:221–222.
[11] Debrunner W. Struktur und Funktion des menschlichen Herzbeutels. Z Anat Entwicklungsgesch. 1956;119(6):512–537.
[12] Carlson MB. Human Embryology and Developmental Biology. St Louis, MO: Mosby-Year Book, 1994:313–315,317.

4

[13] Blechschmidt E, Gasser RF. Biokinetics and Biodynamics of Human Differentiation. Springfield, IL: Charles Thomas Publishers, 1978:3–9,137,143.

[14] Männer J, Seidl W, Steding G. Correlation between the embryonic head flexures and cardiac development. An experimental study in chick embryos. Anat Embryol (Berl). 1993;188(3):269–285.

[15] Emmanouil-Nikoloussi EN, et al. Anterior neural tube malformations induced after all-trans-retinoic acid administration in white rat embryos. I. Macroscopic observations. Morphologie. 2000;84(264):4–11.

[16] Blechschmidt E. Entwicklungsfunktionelle Untersuchungen an Nervensystem. Z Anat Entwicklungsgesch. 1955;119:112–130.

[17] Swynghedauw B. Molecular mechanisms of myocardial remodeling. Physiol Rev. 1999;79(1):216–219.

[18] Geschwind N, Galaburda AM. Cerebral Lateralization. Cambridge, MA: The MIT Press, 1987:3,18–19,47.

[19] Stites DP, et al. Basic and Clinical Immunology. Los Altos, CA: Lange Medical Publications, 1984:302–303,520.

[20] Savino W, et al. Immunoneuroendocrine connectivity: the paradigm of the thymus-hypothalamus/pituitary axis. Neuroimmunomodulation. 1999;6(1-2): 126–136.

[21] Sari A, et al. Le cerveau au service du corps. Paris, France: Sciences et Avenir, 1991:55–61.

[22] De Mello-Coelho V, et al. Role of prolactin and growth hormon on thymus physiology. Dev. Immunol. 1998;6(3-4):317–323.

[23] Grenier B, Fold F. Développement et maladies de l'enfant. France: Masson, 1986:331–351.

[24] Blechschmidt E. Anatomie und Ontogenese des Menschen. Heidelberg, Germany: Quelle und Meyer, 1978:55–66.

[25] Korr I. The Physiological Basis of Osteopathic Medicine. Sevierville, TN: Insight Publishing Co, 1982:21–37.

[26] Wolf S. The stomach's link to the brain. Fed Proc. 1985;44(14):2889–2894.

[27] Grundy D, et al. Gastrointestinal Neurophysiology. Kent, United Kingdom: Baillère-Tindall, 1986:17,29–30.

[28] Rehfeld JF. The new biology of gastrointestinal hormones. Physiol Rev. 1998;78(4):1087–1108.

[29] Gitnick GL, et al. Current Gastroenterology. Hoboken, NJ: Wiley Medical Publication, 1983:183.

[30] Nilsson C, et al. Effects of vasoactive intestinal polypeptide on choroid plexus blood flow and cerebrospinal fluid production. Prog Brain Res. 1992;91:445–449.

[31] Bengmark S, ed. The Peritoneum and Peritoneal Access. London, United Kingdom: Wright, 1989:112,117.

[32] Aube A-C, et al. Inflammation et motricité intestinale. Gastroenterol Clin Biol. 1998;22:509.

[33] Harnsberger HR. Handbook of Head and Neck Imaging. St Louis, MO: Mosby-Year Book, 1995:4–119.

[34] Dobbie JW, et al. New concepts in molecular biology an ultrastructural pathology of the peritoneum: their significance for peritoneal dialysis. Am J Kidney Dis. 1990;15(2):97–107.

[35] Colangelo G. Paediatric osteopathy for children with hyperactivity and behavioural problems. International Conference on Pediatrics; 2000; Utrecht, Netherlands.

[36] Bloomfield GL, et al. Effects of increased intra-abdominal pressure upon intracranial and cerebral perfusion pressure before and after volume expansion. J Trauma. 1996;40(6):936–941.

[37] Vandervert L. The fractal maximum-power. In: Mac Cormac E, Stamenov MI, eds. Fractals of Brain, Fractals of Mind: In Search of a Symmetry Bond. Amsterdam, Netherlands: John Benjamins Publishing Company, 1996.

CHAPTER

5

The importance of tissue integrity in the metabolic field

5.1 The peritoneum, the guardian of the abdomen

The faculty of metabolic exchange depends largely upon the integrity of the tissues organizing the metabolic field of the gut and its annexes. In fact, each visceral lesion could be conceived of as resulting from an aggression upon the supporting tissue and the specialized tissue of exchange. Another consequence of this intimate interaction between the metabolic function and the structuring function of tissue might be that physiological disturbances are automatically reflected upon the metabolic and structuring levels and vice versa. Structure, function, and form are most intimately related at the visceral level. A minute feedback exists between the tissue and the organ, creating compensatory mechanisms of interaction that display local and distant patterns of changed physiology, governed by neurovegetative, vascular, and endocrine adaptations.

When we consider simple, reversible compensations at the abdominal level, two major actors might interfere. The vascular bed initially creates local adaptations, which later will be organized in a more generalized adaptation pattern, induced by released circulating cytokines and hormonal substances (eg, endopeptides, prostaglandins). The same pattern can be discovered in the organization of the neural field, in which local patterns are initially governed by the enteric nervous system (ENS) and later integrated in the central nervous system (CNS). If the local disturbance is not resolved very early, a more generalized physical adaptation can be observed, induced by an altered vascular tonus (vascular reflex) and an altered nervous tonus (nervous reflex)—in other words, increased sympathetic tonus and vagal tonus.

Each tissue lesion displays two sequences:

- First, an edema appears, expressing the more reversible time of the dysfunction (ie, edema could be a defense phase of the tissue or the organ).
- Thereafter, a more irreversible phase appears, in which the tissue increasingly retracts by organizing a state of fibrosis.

Such conditions as fixation, mobility, swelling, and retraction of tissues and organs are precious tools for the practitioner, indicating the degree of urgency for interfering with a specific pathological state. Fascial techniques can be applied punctually and in a direct, corrective manner, or they may follow changing physiological phases of expansion and retraction to guide the tissue and organ to a point of physiological reintegration of its own vital forces.

In osteopathy, this point is described as a "balanced point of reciprocal tension." In some way, the osteopath needs to ascertain that, before normalizing a specific organ dysfunction, the major arterial, venous, and lymphatic passageways between body compartments are free. The laws of exchange and metabolic equilibrium at the abdominal level are mainly governed by fluid and electrolyte exchangeability. Even the patterns of mobility and motility of organs and organizing tissues are largely dependent upon these same laws. No wonder that certain body fluids are kept within a narrow margin of constancy by specialized tissues (ie, cerebrospinal fluid, pericardial fluid, peritoneal fluid). For the cardiopulmonary system and the visceral sphere, most of these fluid alterations are governed by one and the same tissue specialization.

The mesothelial cells of the pleurae and the peritoneum display similar properties of secretion and absorption. Their common origin—from the lateral layer of the mesoderm,[1] the common pleuroperitoneum—not only explains their similarity in function,

---

[1] This is the common origin of the somatopleura and splanchnopleura, which envelop the endocoelomic cavity.

but it also underlines the narrow relationship existing between the thoracic level and the abdominal level to organize a mutual equilibrium.

The intrathoracic pressure and abdominal pressure can be defined as the protagonists of body homeostasis because they govern the laws of exchange of fluids and gases. The physical aspects of the more minute levels of exchange are based on Starling forces. The Donnan effect [1] (also called Gibbs-Donnan equilibrium) reduces much of the therapeutic act to an attempt at restoring arterial-venous-lymphatic passageways. The integrity of the abdominal pressure can be evaluated by well-described manual techniques, serving as a major indication for organizing the therapeutic act of the osteopath. [2]

The main objective is to restore an equilibrated state of fluid exchange between the cardiopulmonary level and the abdominal level. The therapeutic maneuvers used to do so are simple and based upon the physical and biochemical laws of exchange. [3] The osteopath who succeeds in equilibrating both pressures probably understands the mechanics by which tissue and fluid cooperate to create this intrinsic state of physiology. In some cases, physiology can be sufficiently restored by normalizing pressure. In other cases, one needs to treat tissue lesions in a more direct approach to create the possibility of restoring normal abdominal pressure.

One can conceive of the peritoneum as an almost independent organ that displays different properties.

- It displays mechanical properties by *permitting gliding movements of the intraperitoneal and retroperitoneal organs.*
- It provides the anatomical space in which each organ functions in its proper biochemical and biomechanical environment.
- It organizes local and more generalized reaction patterns based upon metabolic and defensive stimuli.[2]
- It represents the chemical-mechanical guardian of visceral integrity, and it functions as a homeostatic go-between.

The creation of the different recesses, organized during embryological rotation of the peritoneal sac, and

the reintegration of the physiological hernia from the umbilical cord into the endocoelomic cavity are important landmarks in structuring the mechanical environment of the organs.[3] [4] They constitute the initial *space-time visceromatrix* of the pleura-cardio-visceral space, analogous to the space-time neuromatrix of the brain and the skull (see chapter 4).

Space is an essential element in creating the necessary parameters to allow normal and organized mobility of the intraperitoneal environment. [5] Not only is the intraperitoneal mobility important in sustaining physiology, but the harmonious mechanical exchange with the subperitoneal space and the retroperitoneal space is based upon reciprocal gliding movements. The subperitoneal space (or the inter-parieto-visceral space) is used as a supportive, gliding plane for the parietal peritoneum.

The lateroconal fasciae seem to play an elementary role in transmitting mechanical forces to the perirenal fascial cones and can be conceived of as a "fascial articulation" between the peritoneum and the retroperitoneum. [6] The kidneys, for example, are held in position not only through the attachments of the renal fascia to the diaphragm, vertebrae, dorsal musculature, and renal pedicle, but also through the effect of the intraabdominal pressure on the renal fossa. [7]

It is now known that the peritoneal canals are phylogenetically older than the pronephric and mesonephric segmental tubes and ducts. In tracing the evolutionary changes of the coelomic cavity from lower life forms to higher vertebrates, one can follow its development as an excretory organ, as part of the reproductive system, and as a lymph reservoir. One of the more challenging concepts of the recent reappraisal of comparative anatomy and physiology of the splanchnocoel is the suggestion that the peritoneal cavity in humans, when provided with an artificial pore, is capable of recapitulating its original excretory function. [8]

Many waste products, including dead mesothelial cells, microbial remnants, and inflammatory fluids,

---

[2] The peritoneum is probably the oldest excretory membrane of the whole body.

[3] As part of the normal developmental pattern, the gastrointestinal trace, during the seventh gestational week, begins its rotation, and the extracoelomic midgut withdraws to the abdominal cavity. This withdrawal is complete in the tenth week of embryonic life. Variations of this normal mechanism are probably responsible for the accessory peritoneal membrane, resulting in encapsulation.

are transported by a properly functioning lymphatic pathway system. The traject followed by this pathway system is orientated toward the submesocolic space, to be collected in the pelvic subperitoneal space and conveyed toward the right and left subphrenic space by way of the laterocolic fossae. [9]

- Another important feature of the peritoneum is the fact that it creates a slippery surface, over which the abdominal viscera can freely glide. The peritoneum can be thought of as *a fluid-secreting surface* that sustains the proper physiology of the imbedded organs. This suggests that the epithelium of the peritoneum creates a lubricated environment consisting of a few milliliters of viscous liquid that constantly regenerates.[4] This liquid contains water, electrolytes, and a mixture of interstitial fluid from adjacent organs and blood plasma.

Furthermore, one should know that the peritoneal membrane is capable not only of minimal fluid secretion, but also of creating a negative electrical field in which adjacent membranes in the peritoneal cavity stay separated from each other. In this way, serosal adhesion[5] is prevented. [10]

As we have previously mentioned, the complete peritoneal cavity acts as a gliding surface for organs, created by space-building processes (recesses) and continuous secretion of peritoneal fluid. Even the subperitoneal space functions as a gliding plane between the fascia parietalis and the fascia subperitonealis. [7]

- Mechanical friction executed by the gliding planes of the serosal membranes or by compressive forces originating from distended organs, together with chemical stimulation by neurotransmitters or strict hormonal messaging, are all capable of activating another feature of this peritoneal covering. The mesothelial cells display underestimated similarities in their fine structure with

pneumocyte 2 cells in the lungs. Both types of cells contain specific lamellar bodies that indicate a significant biosynthetic activity. Evidence that *the mesothelium might be capable of secretory activity* was detected in the abundance of rough endoplasmic reticulum (➤ Fig. 5.1).

With the detection of phosphatidylcholine in the dialysis effluent during transperitoneal dialysis procedures, it was assumed that the mesothelium might be involved in the synthesis of a surfactantlike substance. These surfactant phospholipids are contained in membrane-limited vesicles of various sizes. Hjelle J.T., et al termed these vesicles "surfactosomes." These surfactosomes seem to be present in both intra- and extracellular substances. [11] Dobbie J.W. and Lloyd J.K. [12] found structural and functional similarities between surfactosomes secreted by mesothelial cells of the peritoneum and those secreted by type II pneumocytes (➤ Fig. 5.2).

- Also interesting is the observation that, by the same laws of friction, mechanical stimulation, and biochemical activity, the mesothelial cells are capable of *liberating and favoring production of different types of prostaglandins (PG's)*. [13]

These prostanoids[6] display tissue-protecting features, as well as inflammation-facilitating capabilities. Other prostanoids interfere directly with the

---

[4] The peritoneal cavity contains about 100 mL of fluid. Capillaries participate in the transperitoneal exchange of the fluids and the solutes.

[5] A substance secreted by the mesothelial surface has corresponding properties with these sialomucin substances. The biochemical properties of membrane-associated silaomucin are such that its strong and abundant negative charges produce repulsive forces between facing normal surfaces. This may contribute to prevention of serosal adhesion and reduction of friction during movement of organs. [10]

---

[6] These fatty acids are segregated from membrane phospholipids by phospholipase A2 in response to various physiological and pathophysiological stimuli. They are converted to various prostanoids by sequential action of cyclooxygenase and the respective synthases. Prostanoids thus formed are released outside of the cells immediately after synthesis. Most of the prostaglandins are chemically unstable and are degraded into inactive products under physiological conditions, with half-lives of 30 seconds to a few minutes. They work locally, acting only near the site of their production. Prostanoids exert a variety of actions:
- relaxation of various types of smooth muscles
- modulation of neuronal activity, inhibiting or stimulating neurotransmitter release
- sensitizing sensory fibers to noxious stimuli
- sleep induction and fever generation
- regulation of secretion and motility in the gastrointestinal tract, as well as transport of ions and water in the kidney
- participating in apoptosis, cell differentiation, and oncogenesis
- regulation of the activity of blood platelets, both positively and negatively
- participation in vascular homeostasis and hemostasis.

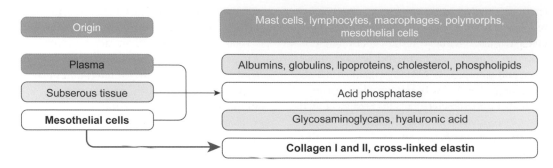

Fig. 5.1 The constellation of peritoneal fluid and its subsequent molecular components

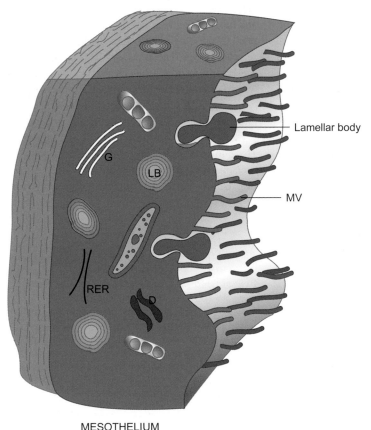

Secretion and absorption of lamellar bodies

MESOTHELIUM

Fig. 5.2 The segregation of a lamellar body at the peritoneal surface and the subsequent secretion of a surfactosome

vascular beds through the activity of other categories of tissue hormones, specifically thromboxanes and prostacyclins. [14]

It is important for the osteopath to understand that physical laws of friction, compression, and hydrostatic exchange govern a great deal of peritoneal and intraperitoneal physiology. The osteopath possesses direct access to the peritoneum by abdominal palpation. Through this access, the osteopath can exert specific pressures on particular anatomical places, which may react with pure tissue reaction patterns or with more complex patterns combining vascular, neurological, and tissue reactions.

- *An elastic lamina sustains most of the mechanical adaptation capabilities of the peritoneum upon mechanical stimuli.* This lamina elastica peritonei (LEP) is a little-known component of the peritoneum, composed of a network of elastic fibers situated immediately beneath the basement membrane of the peritoneal mesothelium. It is separated from this membrane by a scanty layer of connective tissue, poor in collagen fibers. It is particularly common in the areas of organ insertions, indicating that the peritoneal envelopes surrounding the organs can be distended to serve the mobility of the organs and of the complete peritoneal sac. [15]
- The peritoneum's *properties of pain perception and its function as a stretch receptor (localized in the peritoneal meso's)* underline the possibility that the peritoneum is capable of creating local and distant)changes in muscle tonus. [7, 16] It could probably codetermine the vegetative tonus of a great part of the body and interfere with a person's mental and psycho-affective states.
- *Lymphatic dynamics are coordinated by this same peritoneum.* They are guided to the diaphragmatic lacunae formed by stomata in the fascia diaphragmatica of the peritoneum. [17]

Apparently, the whole peritoneal tissue, even the parietal peritoneum, possesses the capability of lymph resorption. There exists a continuity between the peritoneal stomata and the subpleural lymph resorption at the level of their diaphragmatic interface.[7] This contiguous and continuous "articulation" between the subpleural space and the intraperitoneal space indicates that certain inflammatory processes can easily affect two seemingly separated areas and tissues. [18] Negrini D., et al indicate that lymphatic lacunae are more densely distributed on the tendinous peritoneal area than on the pleural one. Continuity between both surfaces has been described. [19]

A symptomatology in the pleural area could indicate a peritoneal suffering or a microbial focus localized at a distance from the actual problem. The peritoneum possesses the remarkable capability of migrating toward the place of infection in order to seal off the focal infection. A special delegate is individualized in the greater omentum, which has been described as one large lymphatic ganglion.

The greater omentum is a special element of defense. It can act as the sentinel of the peritoneal cavity due to two special features. First, it has a mobility that is passive and transmitted. Second, it can fix onto deperitonized surfaces by tropism, and it absorbs by phagocytosis. Being rich in lymphatic structures, it was compared by earlier anatomists to a spread lymph node (Ranvier). [7]

Disturbances in lymph resorption and microbial aggression may profoundly influence the amount of circulating peritoneal fluid. Together with changes in intraperitoneal venous-lymphatic exchange due to portal hypertension or local intraperitoneal vascular obstructions, these disturbances can modify the intra-abdominal pressure.

This subject will be explained later in the text.

- When studying the *anatomical and embryological relationships of the peritoneum,* one could observe that the peritoneum not only serves as a tissue for strongly attaching the organs to the posterior wall of the abdomen, but it also stabilizes the retroperitoneal compartments.

The perirenal fasciae display a common origin with the intraperitoneal mesos, especially the fascia of Toldt on both sides of the peritoneal cavity. [20, 21] The lateroconal fasciae are said to directly stabilize the position of both kidneys. We might propose that in the anatomical insertions of the peritoneal mesos, a great deal of the functionality of the peritoneum as a biomechanical tool is included, along with part of the embryological history. As a biomechanical interface, it serves to stabilize intraperitoneal and retroperitoneal organs.

- Part of *the biomechanical role of the peritoneum* is supported by the intraperitoneal pressure, which helps to maintain normal kidney position,[8]

---

[7] The constant movement of the diaphragm modulates the size of the lymphatic lacunae and stomata. This, coupled with the pressure differential between the abdomen and the thorax, provides a constant upward movement of fluid within the peritoneal cavity (cfr. Bengmark S. *The Peritoneum and Peritoneal Access.* p.75).

---

[8] Feldberg. Computed Tomography of the Retroperitoneum. pp.17–19.

intestinal positioning and intraglandular (hepatic, splenic) pressure values necessary for metabolic and ionic exchange. A normal fluid exchange and mechanics between different intestinal compartments guarantees the position and metabolic processing of the digestive compartment.

- In regard to the reciprocal interference between the intraperitoneal and retroperitoneal compartments, one could suppose that during embryological evolution and fetal and postnatal stabilization of these two compartments, there must have been an intimate and reciprocal mechanical and morphodynamic exchange.

- The anatomy of the lateroconal fasciae and the positions of the organs could suggest a kind of embryologic and morphodynamic fate-mapping that is dependent upon the genetic landscape and the dynamic interferences between two developing fields.

- Even if one accepts an "ascensus renis" (an ascent of the kidneys at the retroperitoneal level), one should consider the 270° rotation of the peritoneal sac and its content as a major co-organizer of the final placement of the kidneys near the diaphragm.

- These considerations mean that an incomplete rotation or an exaggerated rotation of the gut could interfere with the final placement of both kidneys.

- The anatomic topography is different for the right and left kidneys, with the right one normally positioned bit lower than the left one. This is surely related to the volume and weight of the liver at the right site. However, it could also be a consequence of the final insertion of the peritoneal sac on the posterior parts of the parietal peritoneum.

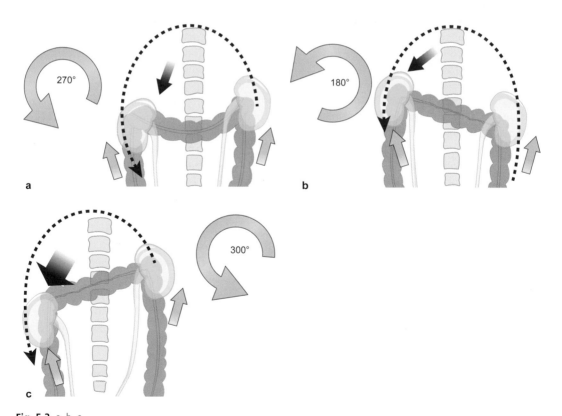

Fig. 5.3 a, b, c
Positioning of the right and left kidneys is dependent upon positioning of the peritoneal sac and its contents, especially the colon.
a: Normal rotation of the colon cadre.
b: Abnormal rotation of the colon cadre: <270°.
c: Abnormal rotation of the colon cadre: >270°.

- The lateroconal fasciae are final landmarks indicating the balanced exchange between the intraperitoneal and extraperitoneal fasciae.
- Different positions of the two kidneys could depend on the complete or incomplete rotation of the abdominal content, as one can see in the figures (➤ Fig. 5.3a, ➤ Fig. 5.3b, ➤ Fig. 5.3c).

For the osteopath, it is important to know about these morphodynamic processes, because they can alter the interpretation of the diagnostic schemes found at the level of the abdomen. If the osteopath finds a kidney descent of second degree or third degree, he or she should ask if the kidney has really sunk down or if the kidney couldn't ascend due to insufficient exchange between the intra- and extraperitoneal cavities.

The kind of treatment provided depends upon this differential diagnosis, which has a direct relation to the morphodynamic histories of these compartments. The tissue memory intrinsically related to these biodynamic processes will express a pattern that is different from the normal physiological ascent and descent of the kidney. The same observation is true for the intraperitoneal landscape.

In addition, the final position of an organ is dependent upon the rotational pattern of the whole peritoneal sac—especially the position of the kidneys and the perirenal fasciae. One should also take into account the rule of holism and the functional interrelationship between different body compartments. This paragraph could function as a caveat for the osteopath to *not be too premature* in diagnosis. Rather, the possibility of a morphodynamic immature or incomplete pattern of organogenesis should be considered.

5.2 Abdominal pressure and its role in the hemodynamic and mechanical organization of digestive physiology

One can see that multiple factors influence the variability of *abdominal pressure*. External pressure of the abdominal wall, diaphragmatic pressure, changes in posture, gas content of the viscera, and fluid exchan-

ges in the venous-lymphatic anastomoses, governed by the physiology of portal pressure, all maintain abdominal pressure in the safety range of 5 to 7.5 mmHg. The peritoneal fluid is minimal in its effects, and its production involves hydrostatic and osmotic pressure. The secreted interstitial fluid accounts for a maximum amount of 100 mL. Nevertheless, the interstitial fluid is positively correlated with changes in abdominal pressure. The serous cavity in males contains almost no fluid. Only females display variations of peritoneal fluid that depend upon cyclic and bacterial changes in the surroundings of the urogenital apparatus.[9] [22]

Major changes in abdominal pressure seem to be correlated with fluctuations of lymph production and absorption in and around the peritoneal cavity. The liver and spleen play a major role in determining exudate quantities generated during their major metabolic phases. The gut and pancreas also can influence changes in fluid quantity during digestive phases. The liver seems to be particularly capable of mastering generation of raised abdominal pressure. Such theories as the overflow and underfill concepts underline the subtle role that the liver plays in governing renine-angiotensine liberation from the kidneys. [23]

Lymphatic unbalance represents a third factor capable of profoundly influencing the abdominal pressure. Concepts about lymphatic rhythmical processes are described later in this chapter.

Disturbance in the rhythmical exchange and progression of lymph is a major co-organizer of digestive pathology and distant symptomatology. In a certain sense, the facility with which an excess of lymph or a stasis of lymph (edema) can occur underlines the subtle equilibrium that exists between arterial-venous-lymphatic vascular fluid exchanges.

A disturbed abdominal pressure can exert two opposed effects upon the underlying physiology:
- Pressure is too high, obliging the intraperitoneal venous capacitance vessels to increase in volume and reducing the circulating volume to and from the heart.
- Alternatively, decreased abdominal pressure reduces most vital exchanges between tissues and

---

[9] Bengmark S. The Peritoneum and Peritoneal Access. p.54.

organs and impedes normal physiology necessary for metabolic equilibrium.

In addition to increased abdominal pressure, the heart will be obliged to adapt its systolic ejection to increased peripheral resistance by changing its rhythm or force of ejection and by altering its end-systolic volume. A substantial part of these adaptive capabilities depends upon the elastic properties of the heart wall and the vessels of the heart base.

As long as the ejection force and volume are not fully adapted to the peripheral resistance, other parts of the body are probably submitted to higher pressure forces than those that sustain their normal physiology. This may be the case even though there is a well-distributed network of pressure-captors dispersed along the most important vascular crossroads (eg, aortic cross, carotid bifurcation).

The brain in particular could be a victim of these high-pressure waves, because the circulating fluid in the brain ventricles needs to be maintained at a normal fluid equilibrium of about 130 mL. This constancy is based on subtle exchanges between blood-brain barriers (eg, Virchow-Robin spaces, plexus choroidei) and CSF-blood barriers (Pacchioni granulations). These subtle exchanges guarantee a homeostatic equilibrium of the biochemical components of the CSF, creating a stable "milieu interne" for the brain function.

This adaptive physiology of fluid pressure exchange and constancy organizes itself by subtle displacements of small volumes of liquor cerebrospinalis (LCS) from the ventricular compartments of the brain to the surrounding subarachnoidal spaces. These parameters of adaptation are defined as "compliance" of the brain. A displacement range of 13 to 16 mL inside the brain spaces is necessary for guaranteeing a normal pressure/volume index of the brain (➤ Fig. 5.4). The subarachnoidal space at the craniocervical junction is the main buffer zone for fluid displacement out of the ventricular part of the brain. Obstruction at that level can raise intracranial pressure, as can several other abnormalities (➤ Fig. 5.5).

Pressure/Volume index

- PVI (pressure/volume index) = the volume added to CSF space that gives a 10-fold rise in pressure.

- PVI of CSF space = 13–16ml.

  Pv (venous intracranial pressure) ≈ Plcs (cerebrospinal fluid intracranial pressure)

- Obstruction to CSF flow at foramen magnum leads to reduced compliance

Fig. 5.4 Compliance of the brain is dependent upon a balance between intracranial venous pressure and cerebrospinal fluid (CSF) pressure.

Compliance of the brain

Compliance enables a volume increase to occur in the intrathecal CNS space without causing a pressure increase, and it corresponds with the amount of venous blood displaced.

- Internal dimensions of CNS bones
- Fontanelles and surgically created bone defects
- Presence of any space-occupying lesion
- CSF volume
- Free flow of CSF around CNS
- Integrity of CNS veins and central venous pressure
- Growth and atrophy of neutral tissue
- Autonomic regulation of blood pressure and flow

Fig. 5.5 Compliance of the brain is also dependent upon a balance between various mechanical and hemodynamic components.

As one can see, the brain possesses its own pressure/volume physiology that depends upon harmonious shifts between intracranial arterial, venous, and LCS pressure. This physiological relationship confirms the intimate dependence of the brain upon cardiac systolic and diastolic pressure shifts and intravascular turbulences.

The pressure wave of the heart travels, in a rather direct way, to the brain over the left carotid artery and, in a more indirect manner, over the right carotid artery. The left carotid forms a direct branching system on the aortic arch, and the right carotid branches off from the brachiocephalic trunk. A deficient absorption[10] of this shock wave could mechanically disturb or irritate brain function.

Changed volume and pressure can also be "sensed," in a subtle way, at the kidney level. These retroperitoneal organs receive about 20% of the cardiac systole and possess rapidly adapting mechanisms to change the renin-angiotensin-aldosterone secretion. By means of this pathway, the kidneys participate at the endocrine homeostatic clock of the body. Their intimate link to the hypothalamic-pituitary-adrenal (HPA) axis implicates them in each level of stress-handling of the body, as well as in each of the phases of cardiovascular adaptations for fluid handling of the heart and its associated regions.

The kidneys create a stable internal "milieu" by monitoring a steady pressure pattern in which glomerular ultrafiltration is elaborated under almost constant pressure values. Changes in glomerular filtration rate and in renal blood flow are expressions of altered internal renal physiology. When physiology is disturbed, the kidneys can adapt by changing the all-round neurological tonus from a sympathetic to a parasympathetic one. But once safety barriers are crossed, the organs become vulnerable to vascular lesions.

Another particularly interesting organ is the spleen. It is well known for the part it plays in the organization of portal hypertension, but little is known or even suggested about its potential role as a shock absorber for the systolic high pressure shocks that arrive at the peritoneum by the way of the celiac trunk.

Its mesothelial origin[11] [24], and its vast reticular construction pattern make the spleen an ideal shock absorber for overly aggressive vascular impulses arriving in an already tensed and aggressed peritoneal envelope. This role might provide an explanation for the assessment that the spleen is sometimes the victim of the portal hypertension and other times the organizer of the portal hypertension.

A decreased abdominal pressure will also organize stases of fluids and create volume-pressure alterations. Decreased pressure means that the fluid exchanges taking place in the peritoneal membranes are impaired and that part of the mechanical function of these fascial compartments may be lost. It is logical that organs and fasciae may diminish fluid return beneath their anatomical localizations when they are displaced, partly because they compress underlying vascular or lymphatic beds and partly because they become progressively fixed to affect a wider area.

The osteopath should always be attentive for expressions of local edema upon an underlying image of abdominal hypopressure or hyperpressure. A congestive image of an organ (showing increased volume or tensed surface) is suggestive for compressive forces exerted on its drainage passages. A diagnosis is made easier if other organs besides the affected one remain well placed and in good shape. Making a diagnosis of normal abdominal pressure or abdominal hyper/hypopressure could be a good expedient for determining the kind of therapeutic maneuvers that should be employed to normalize the diseased state of the patient.

---

[10] A big part of the shock is absorbed by the different fascial envelopes of the brain and by the sigmoid-like trajectories the carotids make in the petro-mastoid parts of temporal bone and in the sinus cavernosus.

[11] Die Milz entsteht als eine Mesenchymverdichtung zwischen beiden Blättern des dorsalen Mesogastriums. Die Milz erhält ihre charakteristische Form schon frühzeitig. Durch die Drehung des Magens kommt es im Bereich der linken Niere zur Verklebung des linken Blattes des Mesogastriums mit dem Peritoneum der dorsalen Bauchwand und damit zur Bildung des Lig. phrenicolienale. Deshalb verläuft beim Erwachsenen die Milzarterie nach links, hinter dem Peritoneum entlang, bis sie dorsal in das Lig. phrenicolienale eintritt. Die Mesenchymzellen der Milzanlage differenzieren sich zum bindegewebigen Stützgerüst, d.h. zum Parenchym der Milz, und bilden auch die Organkapsel.

Abdominal hyperpressure is, in most cases, organized by excessive fluid pressure. This hyperpressure can be caused by an excess of venous portal-caval pressure, lymphatic stasis (leading to ascites), arterial hyperpressure in the liver sinusoids, or hyperpressure in microcapillary exchange within the extracellular matrix of the visceral mesos and fasciae.

We have previously mentioned the detrimental influence that this hyperpressure can have on other organs and fluid equilibrium at a distance. A hepatorenal syndrome (cirrhosis) may lead to chronic renal failure. [25] Increased intra-abdominal pressure may increase intracranial pressure and alter cerebral perfusion. [26, 27] The cardiovascular system may experience changes in peripheral resistance, leading to adaptations in its pressure/volume capacity.

All therapeutic techniques used should be aimed at relieving the local hyperpressure and freeing other organs and fluid exchanges (cranial, cardiovascular, and retroperitoneal). These techniques are mostly hemodynamic maneuvers applied in a rhythmic pattern upon an organ or a specific body area. Fascial molding and myofascial release may precede these maneuvers.

Maneuvers described by W.G. Sutherland [28] for releasing the major diaphragmatic myofascial restriction patterns may be useful for normalizing impediments upon vascular and lymphatic return to the heart base. The pelvic lift, diaphragmatic lift, and cervicothoracic lift maneuvers are meant to relieve the fascial drags that exert impeding influence upon normal physiology. The abdominal hemodynamic maneuver, as described by other authors [2, 3] also deserves great attention and should be taught to every osteopathic student as a preparatory maneuver for re-equilibrating normal pressure patterns in the whole body.

Normal movements, such as respiratory diaphragmatic excursions or peristaltic intestinal mobility, increase pressure in the intraperitoneal area and support fluid absorption and macromolecule absorption at the level of lymphatic vessels. These movements increase the exchange surface between the peritoneal tissue and the residing liquid volume in the peritoneal sac. A three-pore model has been described by B. Rippe by which lymphatic vessels, as well as the interstitial tissue of the peritoneum, should be able to absorb small and large molecules out of the intraperitoneal fluid.[12] [29]

By studying the abdominal hemodynamic maneuver, we note that the practitioner directly increases the abdominal pressure by applying a physical force upon the abdomen. It has been described that an increase in abdominal pressure (in the range of normality: <15 mmHg) also promotes the exchange capabilities between the peritoneal surface and the peritoneal fluid. An increase in fluid absorption and in macromolecule absorption has been verified. Those authors suggest that a high intraperitoneal pressure is associated with an increased lymphatic absorption from the peritoneal cavity. [30, 31]

Another possible effect of physical application of compressive forces to the abdomen is that some vaso-active substances are released, which, even at a distance, might change vascular exchange. It is well known that vasoactive intestinal polypeptide (VIP), peptide histidine isoleucine (PHI), and neuropeptide Y enhance noradrenaline release from sympathetic nerves in the choroid plexus. [32] Local intraperitoneal sensitivity to mechanical stimuli may enhance VIP-release and modify the vascular beds of the peritoneum, the viscera, and their intimate physiology. Thus, it is not astonishing that these circulating substances may reach other areas of the body and interfere with the local bloodstream.

The hemodynamic maneuver seems to interfere well with the arterial-venous-lymphatic exchange units of the visceral domain. Based on this perspective, it is useful to remember some physical and biomechanical factors that are active and interactive during normal lymph progression.

- The integrity of physiological and biochemical processes in organs, articulations, or tissues is based upon arterial-venous-lymphatic exchanges, which are most powerful in the microcirculatory vascular beds (arterioles, micro-arterioles, and their direct venous and lymphatic environment).

---

[12] The author mentions:
- ultrasmall pores of 3–4 A (transcellular water channels)
- small pores of 40–50 A (interendothelial clefts)
- large pores of 250 A (passageway of macromolecules)

- Each organ possesses such a triple exchange mechanism embedded in a loose mesothelial-connective tissue environment.
- The integrity of this tissue guarantees rhythmical exchange and canalization of the produced lymph. Fixation of the connective tissue will impede the normal production and progression of these fluids.
- The lymph stream is subjected to the effects of gravitation, which interferes with the low-pressure gradient of the stream (0.6 mmHg – 1.5 mmHg) in the peripheral mesothelial-connective exchange areas. Slight local compression or more centralized impediment may organize edema in the area of diminished exchange.
- The intrinsic rhythm of the lymphatic circulation is also supported by the anatomical proximity of most of the major arterial branches, which transmit part of their pulsation and kinetic energy upon their nearest anatomical environment. Impediment of these pulsations by anatomical or

traumatic restrictions will alter the normal interference between the blood and lymph.
- Similarly, the biomechanical and respiratory forces exert a substantial mechanical compressing and decompressing force upon the lymphatic bed.
- Lymphatic stasis could be created in moments of tissue exhaustion, corresponding to major rhythmical changes. "Tissue fatigue" can be caused by changes in daily rhythm, digestive congestive phases, post-infectious phases, stress phases, or even hormonal imbalances. In all these cases, tissue fatigue will be found with a subtle subcutaneous edema that might be accentuated at the level of the major fascial-ligamentous arcs of the body (eg, inguinal, subdiaphragmatic, thoracic inlet).
- The major passage levels for the arterial-venous-lymph stream are defined as "*rhythmic zones of the body*" in the osteopathic vocabulary (➤ Fig. 5.6). Ligamentous-osseous conducts and their direct muscular-fascial environment organize

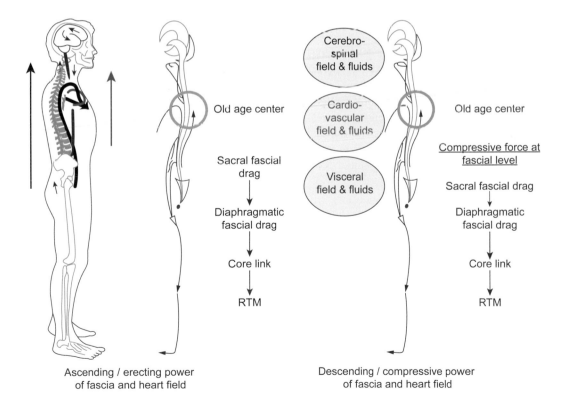

Ascending / erecting power
of fascia and heart field

Descending / compressive power
of fascia and heart field

Fig. 5.6 Erection of the brain is dependent upon erection of the heart, as well as upon proper functioning of the different fields of the body. As an individual grows and matures, the body erects by reciprocal interaction of its structures (eg, heart, intestine, brain) until it is fully ascended. Then, in old age, different fascial drags tend to make the erected individual descend upon these drags.

these rhythmic zones. The great lymphatic axes and clusters of lymphatic ganglions are obliged to cross these critical areas.

The pubic arcs, clavicular arcs, and temporal-zygomatic arcs are excellent examples of passageways for lymphatic circulation. Impediments upon the primary respiratory movement of one of the composing bones of these arcs (pubic bone, clavicle, temporal, zygomatic) can diminish normal lymph progression and create lymph accumulation, such as in the retropharyngeal or submucosal pharyngeal spaces.

• The three major diaphragms of the body are able to disturb normal lymph absorption or progression to the heart in cases of retraction, spasm, or ptosis of their composing parts.
• The deficit of lymph progression can be focused at the mediastinal pleura level or at the cardiopulmonary level proper. When this happens, the urgency for treatment is displaced from a peripheral level to a more centralized level. Edema will be profound, occurring as pulmonary edema.

No further discourse is necessary to demonstrate the importance of integrating maneuvers (eg, hemodynamic abdominal maneuver) into a more complete reasoning about possible causes of local congestion. Every osteopath should possess enough screening tests to assure complete liberty of the major fascial transit areas for fluid progression—or to indicate subtle fixation of some of these key points.

5.3 Destabilization of the anatomical environment of the gut

It could be interesting to examine the hypothesis that a destabilization of the anatomical framework of the gut interferes with normal physiology of the intestine.

Late in the nineteenth century, some well-known physicians proposed that the loss of static of the mechanical environment of the gut could be the origin of onset disease. Is it a coincidence that at about the same time, individuals such as A.T. Still (in the United States) and F. Glénard (in Europe) described the mechanical and pathological implications of a loss of mobility or of a change in anatomical emplacement of parts of the gut? They considered hyper/hypomobility, ptosis, or fibrosis of the viscera as particularly important for the integrity of the anatomical part itself and for its immediate environment.

F. Glénard (1848–1920) has been a major source of inspiration for the further development of the visceral osteopathic concept in Europe. He underlined the importance of hepatic metabolism as a major organizer of disease or health. Glénard introduced the notion of "hépatisme"[13] and "diathèse hépatique" [12] in his 1899 manuscript, Les ptoses viscérales. It was in this manuscript that he mentioned the functional independence of the three major hepatic lobes.

Terms such as gastroptosis, enteroptosis, and splanchnoptosis were meticulously described by Glénard, who defined them by diagnostic particularities found during abdominal palpation. Gastroptosis as a diagnosis could be presumed when borborygmus is heard or manually elicited during manipulation of the proximal part of the gut. Splanchnoptosis could be supposed when a "small pre-aortic tumefaction" transmits the aortic pulsation at the superficies of the abdomen, as detected visually or during light superficial palpation of the abdomen.

An excessively mobile liver palpated during the alternating respiratory cycles is a reliable indicator of hepatoptosis. The term "diathesis," defined as a pre-established disposition to certain forms of disease, is not, in the opinion of Glénard, the only cause for illness. Rather, mechanical factors, such as hyper/hypomobility, form an important aspect of the predisposing arsenal to pathology. In a view of Glénard that is particularly applicable to the visceral domain, the hepatic blood vessels, which are involved in anoxic vasoconstriction organized by catecholamines, are the structures that are most disturbed in the hyperoxidation process by action of the glycocorticoids.

---

13 "Hépatisme, diathèse hépatique" were terms used to indicate the pathological states of the gut or the whole metabolism, determined by altered states of hepatic physiology.

The visceral lesion organized by one of these two possibilities **(hyper/hypomobility or the vascular lesion)** reflects a general change in mechanical parameters of the organ or visceral domain.

Glénard underlines—in agreement with R. Leriche, his contemporary—the importance of the vitality of tissue and the role of capillaries and the nervous systems (central, autonomic, and enteric) in the etiology of pathology. For Glénard, two possible origins of disease could be described as:

- an alteration in nervous activity—that is, the nervous circuitry serving a particular anatomical and visceral domain
- a vascular dysfunction, as was extensively described by Laborit. [12]

A definition of the osteopathic visceral lesion, following the concepts of Glénard, could be phrased as: *a loss or diminution of mobility of an organ and its related tissue that becomes fixed in time and well integrated into the body functioning.*

The notion of time plays an important role in the proper understanding of the lesion—meaning that we not only have to suppress the causes of the dysfunction, but we also have to pay attention to the lesion itself. The tissue and the organ may contain information that is no longer related with the cause but is related with the time the lesion was fixed. Particular movements, a specific pattern of rhythm, an altered motility, or the density of a tissue are all strong indicators of a time pattern interfering with the actual time-space experience of the individual.

Every osteopathic lesion depends upon two types of factors, which are the main time-associated components of the destabilizing momentum of physiology.

- There are gravitational factors with which the individual is not able to cope or to integrate in normal physiology. The abdomen and the organs are submitted to the forces of gravity, against which they defend themselves through the interplay of intramural pressure changes (turgor) and tissue vitality. Thoracic-pulmonary pressure changes will frequently be preceded by, or they may induce, subtle changes in abdominal pressure equilibrium. The whole physiologic interchange will be expressed in an altered relation between abdominal contents and the abdominal wall as a recipient.
- There are connective tissue factors, which, in a pathological state, create a loss of extensibility,

contractility, or elasticity. In such cases, the extracellular and cellular milieu have been deeply altered in their biological and histological components. Vascular troubles can be elicited either by vasomotor phenomena or by axon reflex, which alter the vital field of the supporting tissue and its organ.

Time permits us to make a distinction between a simple phenomenon and a genuine lesion. Sclerosis, dehydration, or loss of antigravitational force are strong indicators of a deeper-lying lesion.

The parameters that permit us to recognize the osteopathic lesion are multiple. There are mechanical parameters that have been used in classical abdominal palpation, and these remain very useful to the osteopath for definition of the visceral lesion.

- *Changes in volume* are the first indication of an altered physiological state. A. Brunnel [33] refers to Sigaud and Thooris, who offered a valuable observation about the changes in form of the intestine: *"Phases of dilatation of the intestine are most of the time primary and reversible. It is a proof that tissues defend themselves energetically. On the contrary, phases of retraction and fibrosis are most of the time terminal and irreversible."*

Every physiological alteration of the gut seems to display two phases:

- There is a dilatation phase, in which the wall of the gut is stretched but tries to restore normal form using all possible reflex patterns appropriate to its metabolic field. For example, chemosensitive and mechanosensitive reflex patterns could be conceived of as being appropriate to the endocrine, paracrine, and neurocrine reaction patterns of the gut. However, they are also probably part of the intricate defense mechanism that the gut wall uses against excessive stresses. The sooner the dilatation phase is restored to normal, the less the tissue is impregnated with an altered a-physiological state of functioning.
- There is a retraction phase, which indicates a definitive changed state of the gut.

An excessively long-lasting dilatation of the gut wall probably exceeds the adaptation capabilities of the intrinsic tissues (serosa, longitudinal and circular muscle layers, mucosa, submucosa) and creates an inflammatory reaction pattern of the tissue by liberating a diversity of prostaglandins and cytokines. If the inflammatory state lasts too long, a retraction pattern is organized, leading to fibrosis.

It is clear that the osteopath has to be aware of these subtle changes so that techniques can be adapted to the altered physiological state of the tissue. For example, direct techniques used upon an inflamed colon could worsen the condition, whereas indirect techniques could gently increase a normal physiological state. Perhaps this was the reason that W.G. Sutherland cautioned against an excessively aggressive approach to the abdomen.[14] Direct techniques seem more appropriate to stimulate and free densified or retracted tissues or organs.

- *Changes in form* can be interpreted in two ways:
  - A form that is modified from within expresses a real lesion.
  - A form that is modified from the exterior usually expresses a phenomenon. For example, something can compress or deform an organ without the organ being in a diseased state.
- *Changes in relief* are indicative of inner abdominal or intestinal pressure changes.
- *Changes in density* are indicative of the probability that the noble cells and vascular tree of an organ are going to be compressed, depending upon the degree of hardness and extent of the density.
- *Changes in position* of an organ are due to intrinsic predisposing factors (eg, dolichocolon) or are dependent upon changes in extrinsic factors (eg, organ contiguity, pressure, anatomical relationship). It is not clear whether a change in position elicits a change in intrinsic function of the organ [34], but it is realistic to suppose that a change in position of an organ could compress the vital field of other organs or its own neurovascular route.
- *Loss of mobility* of a specific organ or digestive area could be an effect of fibrosis or a cause for altered intrinsic physiology. We can state that every organ possesses its own movement and basic rhythmical pattern.

Pathology usually starts progressively, though not necessarily slowly, by displaying an altered pattern of energy distribution. Later in the disease process, one will find functional signs representing the underlying cause. Eventually, the disease will appear in its definitive form.

Loss of energy or changes in energy patterns can be interpreted as an expression of the fact that the body can no longer assure its own homeostatic level. The functional signs indicate an attempt at adaptation to the changes, which have started to enter the tissue as changes in density, irrigation, warmth, or hyper/hypomobility.

The lesion itself may appear gradually or suddenly, but the precursor sign of the lesion is always a change in volume of the tissue or organ. The organ may feel initially like a full rubber ball. Congestion of the tissue or organ is the first sign that should remind the therapist of the possibility of disease. Later during the disease process, the organ may display a diminished volume due to fibrosis and retraction of its supporting tissues. Most intestinal lesions are the result of vascular imbalance, and Dr. Still knew that *the circulatory lesion originated in the belly.*

When there is a need for slowing down normal circulation, the intra-abdominal venous blood circuit starts functioning as a "spare tank" that intimately cooperates with the cardiovascular system to guarantee irrigation of all tissues and organs. This venous spare tank can contain almost two-thirds of the total circulating blood volume.

Both sudden and gradual changes in the volume of an organ or its fascial environment are able to stress normal mobility and fixation expedients, inducing gradual alteration of the tissue integrity of the organ. Sooner or later, the organ will display altered features in its intimate physiology. The first signs of this could be rather minor alterations, such as skin irritations or densifications caused by lack of absorption of vital vitamins.

In most cases, one could postulate that a general increase in volume of the intestine, if not quickly resolved, will alter the normal anatomical and physiological relation between the organ and its environment. If this condition persists for a long period, it will result in a general destabilization of the digestive sphere. This progression will lead to a state of enteroptosis.

---

[14] Have a keen and gentle approach to the abdomen and its contents. (W.G. Sutherland)

REFERENCES

[1] Kayser C. Physiology. Paris, France: Flammarion, 1970:256–257.

[2] Weischenk J. Traité d'ostepathie viscérale. Vol 1. Paris, France: Maloîne, 1982.

[3] Vuffray M. La grande manoeuvre abdominale hemodynamique. Lausanne, Switzerland: Ecole Suisse d'Ostéopathie, 1999.

[4] Sayfan J, et al. Peritoneal encapsulation in childhood. Case report, embryologic analysis, and review of literature. Am J Surg. 1979;138(5):725–727.

[5] Feldberg MAM. Computed Tomography of the Retroperitoneum. Leiden, Netherlands: Martinus Nijhoff, 1991:17–19.

[6] Hureau J, et al. The posterior interparietoperitoneal spaces or retroperitoneal spaces. 1: Normal topographic anatomy. J Radiol. 1991;72(2):101–116.

[7] Bengmark S, ed. The Peritoneum and Peritoneal Access. London, United Kingdom: Wright, 1989:5–12.

[8] Dobbie JW. New concepts in molecular biology and ultrastructural pathology of the peritoneum: their significance for peritoneal dialysis. Am J Kidney Dis. 1990:15(2):97–109.

[9] Gore RM, et al. Textbook of Gastrointestinal Radiology. 2nd ed. Philadelphia, PA: W.B. Saunders Co, 1994:2354.

[10] Ohtsuka A, et al. Localization of membrane-associated sialomucin on the free surface of mesothelial cells of the pleura, pericardium, and peritoneum. Histochem Cell Biol. 1997;107(6):441–447.

[11] Hjelle JT, et al. Autosomal recessive polycystic kidney disease: characterization of human peritoneal and cystic cells in vitro. Am J Kidney Dis. 1990;15(2):123–136.

[12] Dobbie JW, Lloyd JK. Mesothelium secretes lamellar bodies in a similar manner to type II pneumocyte secretion of surfactant. Perit Dial Int. 1989;9(3):215–219.

[13] Bengmark S, ed. The Peritoneum and Peritoneal Access. London, United Kingdom: Wright, 1989.

[14] Narumiya S, et al. Prostonoid receptors: structures, properties, and functions. Physiol Rev. 1999;79(4):1193–1226.

[15] Knudsen PJ. The peritoneal elastic lamina. J Anat. 1991;177:41–46.

[16] Kamina P. Abdomen paroi et appareil digestif. Vol 1. Paris, France: Maloîne, 1993.

[17] Bengmark S, ed. The Peritoneum and Peritoneal Access. London, United Kingdom: Wright, 1989:63-65,75,85–90.

[18] Wang NS. The preformed stomas connecting the pleural cavity and the lymphatics in the parietal pleura. Am Rev Respir Dis. 1975;111(1):12–20.

[19] Negrini D, et al. Distribution of diaphragmatic lymphatic lacunae. J Appl Physiol. 1992;72(3):1166–1172.

[20] Feldberg MAM. Computed Tomography of the Retroperitoneum. Leiden, Netherlands: Martinus Nijhoff, 1983:21.

[21] Hureau J, et al. The posterior interparietoperitoneal spaces or retroperitoneal spaces. 1: Normal topographic anatomy. J Radiol. 1991;72(2):101–116.

[22] Koninckx PR, et al. Origin of peritoneal fluid in women: an ovarion exudation product. Br J Obstet Gynaecol. 1980;87(3):177–183.

[23] Köhler H, Meyer KH. Funktionelle Beziehung zwischen Leber und Niere. Dtsch Med Wochenschr. 1988;113(38):1486–1491.

[24] Moore KL. Embryologie. Stuttgart, Germany: Schattauer, 1985:266–267.

[25] Dudley FJ, et al. Hepatorenal syndrome without sodium retention. Hepatology. 1986;6(2):248–251.

[26] Bloomfield GL, et al. Effects of increased intra-abdominal pressure upon intracranial and cerebral perfusion pressure before and after volume expansion. J Trauma. 1996;40(6):936–941.

[27] Bloomfield GL, et al. Elevated intra-abdominal pressure increases plasma renin activity and aldosterone levels. J Trauma. 1997;42(6):997–1004.

[28] Sutherland WG. Teachings in the Science of Osteopathy. Cambridge, MA: Rudra Press, 1990.

[29] Rippe B, Zakaria ER. Lymphatic versus nonlymphatic fluid absorption from the peritoneal cavity as related to the peritoneal ultrafiltration capacity and sieving properties. Blood Purif. 1992;10(3-4):189–202.

[30] Zinc J, Greenway CV. Intraperitoneal pressure in formation and reabsorption of ascites in cats. Am J Physiol. 1977;233(2):H185–H190.

[31] Imholz AL, et al. Effect of an increased intraperitoneal pressure on fluid and solute transport during CAPD. Kidney Intl. 1993;44(5):1078–1085.

[32] Nilsson C, et al. Effects of vasoactive intestinal polypeptide on choroid plexus blood flow and cerebrospinal fluid production. Prog Brain Res. 1992;91:445–449.

[33] Brunnel A. Anatomie et mécanique des viscères abdominaux. Fascicule. 1983;2.

[34] Hamburger J, et al. Néphrologie Urologie. 3rd ed. Paris, France: Flammarion Médicine, 1980:97.

5

CHAPTER

6

The heart as a key point in the osteopathic approach

6.1 Introduction

The heart can be considered as a mobile fulcrum that integrates and orchestrates all of the hemodynamic forces of the body within its inner dynamics. The heart develops as a progressive answer to energy demands of the brain and the rest of the embryo's body. In other words, the development of the heart as a pumping mechanism is related to a progressively increasing need of the embryo's developing brain for nutrients and oxygen. The only organ that can afford this demand is the liver, which integrates and filters the incoming blood of the vitelline and placental circulation. There is also an increase in the volume of the liver in relation to the increasing metabolic needs of the brain.

The heart must respond to the growing metabolic fields of both the brain and the liver. Its change in volume and orientation occurs in response to these two organogenetic events. The heart functions as the concentrated meso of the whole body plan. It is the major go-between in the interplay between information and function, between dynamics and stability.

Therefore, the heart displays great variability in its adaptability to rhythm, pressure, motion, and fluid dynamics. It is not only a dynamic device for guaranteeing blood supply to all body systems, but it intimately participates in the homeostatic maintenance of the body by interfering with endocrine and autonomous adaptations. During its systolic and diastolic phases, it displays a dynamic interplay between extrinsic and intrinsic structures that guarantees its fluent adaptation to peripheral resistance and energy demand.

For the osteopath, it is important to understand how all of these functions have been integrated in a complex pulsating field that is sustained primarily by a fascial environment that simultaneously affords stability and mobility. Furthermore, it is necessary to study the intrinsic and extrinsic interferences that were worked out during embryogenesis and fetal development. For better understanding the functions of the heart, one should know that function relies upon the intrinsic neurophysiology of this organ and upon its dynamic interference with its immediate environment. This environment is built up by the major blood vessels and the mediastinum.

Although the heart seems to be the major housekeeper of the mediastinum, one should not forget that its final emplacement is guided by lung and liver development and by the subsequent changes in fascial organizations of the pleuroperitoneal and peritoneal compartments. It is of major importance for the osteopath to determine how the heart is handling the major fluid and rhythm changes of the body, all in accord with the support provided by the major fascial compartments of the visceropleura. Restrictions in the mediastinal space will automatically interfere with the adaptive capabilities of the heart in its fluid handling, automaticity, and intrinsic motility.

A major part of the heart's physiology is based upon a subtle, progressive adaptation to increasing workload, in which it must constantly reassemble parts of its original segments into newly adaptive and functional compartments. The mature heart can be considered as an assembly of subsequent segments arranged into functional anatomical compartments. Its workload-related functional modification means that the heart adapts to its environment not only by intrinsic changes of its contractile forces and dynamics, but also by changes in form and orientation related to a restrictive fascial environment organized by visceropleural dynamics.

It is evident that all of these transformations are stored as space/time units in the intimate lattice of actin/myosin filaments, in the construction and organization of the heart's four chambers, and in the spatial and structural arrangements of the heart's myocard, endocard, and epicard. The heart not only has an adaptive hemodynamical function, but it adapts itself upon load by relying on integrated patterns during development. In that way, function becomes an actualized state as well as a referential development of potential rhythms and pressure/volume adaptations.

6.2 Developmental milestones

"Cardiac morphogenesis involves intrinsic cellular and molecular interactions, but these must occur against a background of ongoing mechanical function." [1]

From the osteopathic point of view, the main questions concerning the developmental logic of the heart could be worded as follows:

- Does the heart develop solely upon cellular-molecular interactions guided by genetic information?
- Is it guided by mechanical information depending on its intrinsic and extrinsic environment?
- Are early hemodynamic components the major organizing forces that direct the form and function of the heart, in conformity with extrinsic forces resistant to the flow impulses of the embryological bloodstream?

If the heart is organized by intrinsic factors, one should accept that it controls the major part of the hemodynamic physiology because it is essentially independent from its environment. If, by contrast, one accepts that the heart is a part of the whole, then the role of the heart as an integrating organ becomes more evident. In the latter vision, we could conceive of the heart and its pulsation as an "echo" of the peripheral vascular and hemodynamic resistances.

The pulsation of the heart that is perceived when taking a radial pulse (chronotropy) is not only the expression of the rhythm and intrinsic force of the heart pump. It is also a reflection of the dynamic, mechanical response of the heart to the pressure and volume variables of peripheral resistance (inotropy/dromotropy). Such physiological values as "preload" and "after-load" should be interpreted in this context as the intrinsic and extrinsic factors defining the heart dynamics. These physiological values

represent integrative steps in the morphodynamic development of the heart during the subsequent phases of embryologic, fetal, and postnatal adaptation to intrinsic and extrinsic changes in volume and tissue load.

In a certain sense, the heart is constantly adapting to changes in workload and trying to integrate the physiological parameters into biomechanical and biodynamic diversification. It is probable that the heart integrates these parameters as subtle changes in rhythm and contractile force, and that much of the variability of heart rhythm is due to early adaptations of its intrinsic structuring upon the increasing complexity of body physiology. This physiology is an expression of all the biological components needed for guaranteeing homeostasis. It comprises biochemical, bioelectrical, biomolecular, and biomechanical parameters, which have to be balanced in rheodynamical and electrodynamical values. The heart is like a storage place for all these interactions.

During its development from a single tube to a four-chambered organ, the heart gathers information about resistance to rheodynamical ease of fluids throughout the body (and it continues doing so throughout adult life). B. Freeman[1] describes the heart as a commutator that reverses the direction and momentum of the blood current between inflow and outflow. This happens as early as the end of the first month after conception, when the developing heart gathers the incoming volume to expel it toward the periphery. Moreover, the incoming, eddying blood progressively changes the inner texture of the cardiac endothelium.

The stronger the eddylike currents become, the more powerful is the transformation of the cardiac jelly into a specific structure, later known as the trabeculae carneae. One could conceive of this structure as being among the first integrated field memories in which the rhythm and increasing power of life are laid down into a specific anatomy, a type of "geography." The trabeculated regions of the primitive heart chambers are the first indicators of the adaptive and integrative response of the endothelium of the heart

---

1 Blechschmidt E; Freeman B, ed. *The Ontogenetic Basis of Human Anatomy*. Berkeley, CA: North Atlantic Books, 2004:173-175.

to incoming blood flows that vary in volume and pressure. The hemodynamic values depend on the peripheral resistance and the volume that the developing heart has to integrate. Thus, the trabeculated regions form a kind of topographic recording of hemodynamic values within the developing organism.

During its morphogenesis, the heart gathers in its intimate physiology all the data about changes in peripheral needs, governed by the laws of the pressure/volume relationship. It is through this process that the heart becomes able to change its contractility and rhythm to meet all vital needs of the body. The heart takes up all possible space/time units and transforms them step by step into useful adaptive tools for responding to the subtle demands of oxygen supply, hemodynamic force, and fluid exchange.

The intrinsic Ca^2 oscillations in the cardiomyocytes—the intimate relationship between actin/myosin bridges during contraction and relaxation—can be conceived of as subtle quantum devices regulating the intrinsic adaptability of the heart to different frequencies at microtime levels. The hemodynamic microtimes of the eddylike currents support the continuous transformation of heart function throughout the embryologic/fetal period. Finally, the heart becomes able, at birth, to transmit its intrinsic adaptation to flow and resistance in a hemodynamic pattern, guaranteeing antigravitational power.

Microtimes have become macrotimes (beat/pulse and pressure), and these macrotimes simultaneously transmit the secrets of the heart in specific sequences to the periphery. These subtle changes are not always perceived in electrocardiograms, but they can be detected in field exchanges between heart and brain, and the heart and viscera.

It is probable that the heart can transmit subtle changes to the brain by changing the power of its contraction and by changing the vortices in the blood flow arriving in the brain.[2] It is clear that the heart senses qualia at the periphery by subtle volume and pressure receptors in the atria and by chemoreceptors in the atria and auricula (ANP).

All these parameters are meant not only for supporting physiology, but also for informing the heart

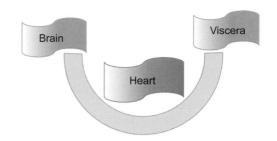

Fig. 6.1 The heart field represents the intermediate field between the brain and the viscera.

about the varying sensitive landscape at the periphery (viscerosensitivity), governed by the autonomic and the neuro-endocrine pathways. Part of this information is related to the way the brain handles emotions, transforming them into viscerotonus. The heart receives and transmits the response of the visceral field upon emotion to the brain and the other homeostatic fields (immune/endocrine fields). By this means, it completes the feedback loop between brain and viscerum and functions as a fulcrum for emotional balance (➤ Fig. 6.1).

6.3 Cellular and tissular origins controlling form and anatomical emplacement of the heart

The tissue component of the embryonic heart displays different origins:

- The atrial-ventricular myocardial tissue arises from a horseshoe-shaped bilateral primordium of the splanchnic mesoderm. Part of this primordium might even belong to the extra-embryonic mesoderm. One could make a distinction between a primary heart field, providing the precursors for most of the left ventricle, and a more ventral field, providing the precursor for the atria and the efferent vessels.[3]

[2] Goncharenko AI. Hemodynamical vortices originate in the heart. *Delphis Journal.* 2003;3:112-116.

[3] Tardy M-M, et al. Embryologie des cloisons du coeur. *Morphologie.* 2013;97:2-11.

- The outflow tract, in its endothelial layer, depends upon components arising from the cephalic and lateral mesoderm (otic placode).
- The major cellular component of the outflow tract is derived from neural crest concentrations in the midotic placode, and it extends to the level of the third somite.

From the earliest development, one can note the intimate relationship that exists between visceral-splanchnic information and heart function. Another remarkable fact is the intrinsic dependence of the major part of the outflow tract upon the information originating in the occipital region. Two different cell populations seem to be important at this level:

- cells migrating out of the upper occipital somites
- cells migrating out of the cranial neural crest in the neighborhood of the otic placode

The looping of the heart also seems to be dependent upon molecular and intrinsic structuring components. The underlying morphological changes seem to depend upon multiple factors:

- the orientation of the constituting microtubules
- the asymmetrically located bundles of actin
- pressure of the cardiac jelly
- changes in the shape of individual myocardial cells.

Local mechanical conditions may participate in orientating and transforming the local mesodermal myocardial primordium. The descent of the pro-enteron, local hemodynamic pressure changes, and early fixations of the heart tube are interfering factors in early embryogenesis. They will be discussed later.

The result of all these interactions is that the heart appears as the first asymmetrical organ of the embryonic body. Are these asymmetries induced by local morphogenetic factors, or are they more a result of interfering asymmetrical biodynamic and biomechanical forces? If the latter is true, this means that the heart, in its inner constellation and orientation, is directly dependent upon its mechanical and hemodynamic environment.

It is likely that many of these factors continue to interfere with heart motion and function during adult life, and they could even be the major cause of dysfunction of this pump when it loses its proper physiology.

We previously mentioned that each structural transformation in the form or tissue of the heart could be considered as a progressive series of memory stacking during morphogenesis. Each of these levels of transformation could alter the subtle dynamics of the heart in its hemodynamic, electrical, or motion components.

6.4 The mesodermal environment of the heart and its importance in the orientation of the heart tube

Apparently the mesodermal environment of the heart influences its rotation and emplacement in two distinct anatomical areas of the early heart tube.

- The outflow tract displays an intimate exchange with the *"mesendodermal anlage"* of the neck organs and the accompanying musculofascial trajectories (sterno-cleido-mastoid muscle, lingual apparatus, thyroid, and thymus). [2] The muscular walls of the outflow tract remain in close relationship with the tissue continuity between the fascias of the pericard and the fascias of the subhyoidal region. There is a kind of electrical continuity between the muscular wall of the heart, the muscular wall of the great outflow arteries (aorta, pulmonary arteries), and the muscles of the subhyoidal region. [3]
- The inflow tract is subjected to the dispatching forces emitted by the developing diaphragm. The major inserting ligaments of the heart are intrinsically related to the diaphragm. Debrunner [4] as early as 1956, described the right, left, and posterior cardiophrenic ligaments (ligamenta cardiophrenica) as the most potent attachment expedients of the heart. Through these attachments, the heart is submitted to the respiratory expansions of the diaphragmatic dome. In fact, these ligamentous attachments display as local reinforcements of the global pleurovisceral fascia.

A number of other textbooks have described the ligaments around the heart sac as rather inconstant, noting that they should be considered as local reinforcements upon mechanical or inflammatory cues needing local adaptation of physiology.

Fetal breathing movement, described as "gasps" starting during the 20th week, seem to be important in orientating the pericard and the epicard envelopes. [5–8] The pull of the diaphragm through sudden contraction participates in activating the elasticity and activity of the myo-epicard.

- Another intimate mesodermal relationship is established by the early pro-enteron as it cooperates during the first phase of the heart descent. When the heart is still situated in the neck region, the proximal gut descends into the pleuroperitoneal cavity and positions the heart bulge in the cephalad part of this same cavity. The descent of the heart also orientates the primal left position of the proximal gut (pro-enteron).
- The later episodes of descent and emplacement are organized by the development of the visceral-abdominal area, especially the liver, and also by the ascent of the head, which becomes more and more mechanically supported by the axial musculoskeletal system. This episode is also referred to as the ascensus of the spinal cord versus the descensus viscerum.

The heart becomes increasingly orientated along a cephalic-caudal axis, and the ventricles become oblong. The descensus cordis probably continues until the age of three years; the apex of the heart is then found in the third or fourth intercostal space. [9]

A series of morphogenetic processes occur after the heart tube has been formed by ventral apposition of two original tubes (or cardiogenic plates) and begins to beat in the vicinity of the anterior splanchic mesoderm at the end of the second week. The induction of the primitive heart at that time is dependent upon endodermal signaling, which orchestrates the differentiation of precardiocytes, which, in turn, migrate toward the cardiogenic plate at the anterior part of the embryo.

Afterward, morphogenetic transformations definitively shape the heart toward its adult form. These transformations are expressed in three major stages of the heart's intrinsic development:
- *Loopings*, displaying proximal, middle, and distal incisures (bent grooves produced by slight lateral and torquing movements of the early segments of the heart tube).

- *Convergence*, also described as a cropping of the heart.
- *Wedging* of the heart, in which the conotruncus and the initial segments of the aorta and pulmonary artery are septated and displaced toward their definitive relation with their respective ventricles. The wedging is specified by a remodeling of the inner curvature of the heart, which is the starting sign for ventricle septation and valve development.

The early looping is characterized by a lateral inflexion of the heart tube, slightly toward the right and bending toward an anterior convexity. This is the C-loop (➤ Fig. 6.2). The later process is organized by a displacement of the conotruncus toward the left and the atrioventricular canal toward the right. The primitive atria will ascend behind the primitive ventricle, and it finally will be fixed behind the left and right ventricles. This is the S-loop (➤ Fig. 6.3).

In the meantime, an intensive reorganization takes place at the inner curvature of the loop. This reorganization will be important for the major transformations at the endocardial and myocardial parts of the heart (endocard cushions, valves, septa). [10] This whole process seems to be organized by the mobile venous part of the early heart tube (primitive inflow segment), which displaces the distal part of the heart tube to the left, posterior, and cephalad.

The sinus venosus probably plays an important role as an organizer of looping and tissue information, though the proximal mesocard could organize the first torque of the arterial segment in a rightward rotation. The sinus venosus could be defined in several ways as a transitional fulcrum—for hemodyamic remodeling, for inductive activity during cardiomyocyte development and migration, for transformation of the epicardial fascial envelope of the primitive heart, and for participation in the emplacement of the sinus node. It concentrates the primordium of the sinoatrial node on the right side of the heart, beneath the right atrium.

One could note that part of the later function of the heart is a rehearsal of mechanical events happening during embryogenesis and fetal maturation. Part of the adult function of the heart could be considered as pure memory—a well organized and repetitive

6

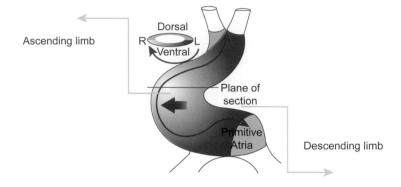

Fig. 6.2 The inner curvature of the heart tube is represented by the C-loop.

multifunctional system of successively integrated dynamical patterns. These patterns are integrated as successive space/time units in all the composing parts of the heart. The heart transforms progressively into a landscape of integrated space/time units. The pericardial sac, for example, integrates in its intimate collagen fiber organization a great part of the original cardiac looping orientation.

Manasec and Monroe [11] mention that this integration process depends partially upon mechanical stimuli, which cause cardiac jelly pressure changes and morphological changes in the orientation of the early pro-enteron. This proximal part of the gut starts to display a predominant convexity to the left in the embryonic pleuromediastinal cavity. [12]

One should not forget that the heart, during its descent, plays an important role in orienting the esophagus to the left, installing a mutual interference during this important biodynamical episode. At the same time, all these factors create changes in elasticity of the myocard through different concentrations in synthesis of myofibrils.

Even the epicard, in its stratum elastico-reticulare and stratum fibrilare, displays a net spatial orientation pattern. A net difference in orientation of elastic and collagenous fibers depends on changing patterns of mechanical stress that the heart underwent during embryogenesis. The orientation of these fibers will play an important role in how the heart handles its preload and prepares itself for systolic motion.

The epicardial fiber pattern for the left ventricle manifests a clear counterclockwise rotation, continuous from the interventricular septum to the apex of the heart. Manifestly, this pattern coincides with the diastolic filling sequence of the left ventricle, and it is used in an opposite way to express systolic contraction. [13] In a certain way, the pericard and the epicard constitute a map of orientated force lines that are organized during organogenesis.

It is interesting to note that many of the epicard cells originate from the serosal layer of the septum transversum (➤ Fig. 6.4). A close relationship between the diaphragm and the peri/epicard should be kept in mind. Epicardial orientation will also be important for determining the pattern of the coronary vascular network.

Two remarkable facts can summarize this chapter:
- The pro-enteron participates in an important way in the orientation and formation of the heart loopings and their subsequent deformations. It interferes with the heart in two ways:
  – partly as an elongating rope ladder around which the heart orientates
  – partly as a passive structure depending upon the dynamics of the heart descent.
- The intrinsic relationship between the heart and the diaphragm is expressed not only by a continuity by fascial-ligamentous attachments, but also by a common origin of the cell population of the epicard and the serosal layer of the diaphragm's centrum tendineum.

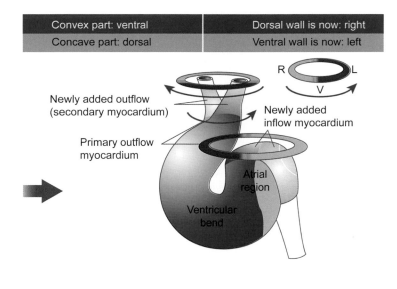

Convex part: ventral	Dorsal wall is now: right
Concave part: dorsal	Ventral wall is now: left

Newly added outflow
(secondary myocardium)

Newly added
inflow myocardium

Primary outflow
myocardium

Atrial
region

Ventricular
bend

Fig. 6.3 The S-loop represents the ascent of the primitive atria, spiraling and ascending behind the ventricular bend and the outflow tract.

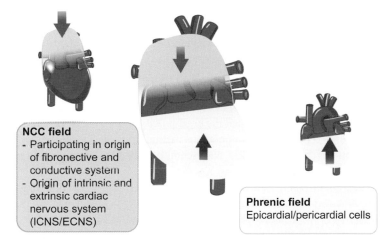

NCC field
- Participating in origin of fibronective and conductive system
- Origin of intrinsic and extrinsic cardiac nervous system (ICNS/ECNS)

Phrenic field
Epicardial/pericardial cells

Fig. 6.4 The neural crest cells (NCC's) form the cranial field of the heart, organized around the cardiac outflow tract. Serosal cells from the septum and the primitive splanchnopleura form the distal field.

Part of the fascial envelope of the heart constitutes a common field between the original splanchnopleura, the septum transversum, and the intrinsic fascial relationship of the heart with its immediate surroundings—esophagus, bronchi, and pleurae. The osteopath has to keep in mind this common origin in evaluating the dynamics of the heart and its effective volume handling.

6.5 Hemodynamic components organizing heart function

It is almost certain that extrinsic factors play an important role in organizing the myofascial environment of the heart. A logical question could be: Is the pumping and pulsating activity of the heart an intrinsic property of the muscle or a consecutive adaptation upon changing hemodynamic and hydrostatic pressure values, inside and outside the heart cavity?

There is an intrinsic electrical activity at the level of the precardiocytes near the end of the second week. This activity will organize a peristaltic interaction of the primitive heart tube with the incoming blood. It is also known that part of the rhythmicity of the heart is transmitted by the venous inflow tract and by cells originating from the original splanchnopleura at that level.

Pressure-volume relationships of the different heart cavities suggest that the heart, after its morphodynamic processing, is rhythmically dependent upon a resting volume and a resting length of its muscle fibers. In this way, it combines its intrinsic contractility with the external load upon which it has to counteract.

Force and rhythm seem to be as much dependent upon external factors as they are upon intrinsic electrical rhythm and muscular contractility. In other words, could it be that the heart is a mesodermal response upon different kinds of pulse-waves originating in other tissues—a response conveyed to the cephalic area by primitive bloodstreams? The early heart placode could be considered as the place where these streams concentrate and flow back to the periphery, thus eliciting a countershock. Therefore, it seems reasonable to believe that the heart pulsation is a response rather than an autonomous rhythm.

In one of his last books, Blechschmidt [14] wrote:*"Die Herzanlage ist zunächst eine Interzellularsubstanz sammelende Gewebsfalte. Je mächtiger das Herz heranwächst, desto mehr führt es, bereits seit der vierten Entwicklungswoche auch zu rhythmischer Tätigkeit befähigt, 'Blut' in erster Linie der Gehirnanlage zu. Das bereits strömende Blut dehnt die Herzwand: Es entsteht ein Dehnungsfeld, in welchem sich die Zellen zu Muskelzellen dilatieren."*[4]

Blechschmidt wrote that the early heart anlage can be conceived of as an "Interzellularsubstanz," a kind of intercellular matrix that progressively displays an epithelial constitution. The heart displays a matrix with epithelial lining between the epiblastic and hypoblastic layers at the frontal part of the embryonic disc. The primitive heart anlage represents a crescentlike structure laid down in front of the notochordal apex. It lies between the future brain field, in front and above, and the endodermal field, behind and beneath. It gives the impression of being a kind of dynamic/plastic fulcrum between two important metabolic fields.

It seems evident that the original nourishing stream of the embryonic body (vitelline and umbilical vessels) orientates the early heart in a right-shift, by which all the important venous systems of the body are orientated to the right (ductus venosus, sinus venosus, vena cava, left vena brachiocephalica, sinus coronarius). This venous "return system" toward the right heart favors the development of the right atrial structure and its direct communication with the left atrium (ostium primum and secundum). Furthermore, it exercises the right ventricle in its future contracting and pumping function.

An identical pattern can be individualized for the arterial organization of the heart. The initial arterial blood flow is organized in a left-shift.

- The fourth branchial arch shunts from the right to the left and builds the aortic arch and the internal carotid artery.
- The creation of the ductus arteriosus is another anatomical adaptation of the early arterial bloodstream to the left. It directs the oxygen-rich blood to the brain, instead of conveying it into the left ventricle and then to the rest of the body.

This proves that the heart is organized upon the energy needs of the young brain, supporting early cerebralization. The direct continuity between the aortic arch and the left internal carotid artery is a functional remnant of this important left-shift.

For the osteopath, it could be very useful to determine how far the heart, in its pericardial environment, is preferentially orientated upon a venous return (right shift) or upon an arterial, systolic outflow system (left shift). Seated at the head of the patient, the osteopath can test the base of the heart by laying his or her right hand upon the upper and middle mediastinum, with the palm directed along the main axis of the heart (the apex of the heart being situated in the fifth intercostal space at the left side of the sternum). The digits touch the area of the apical shock, and the proximal part is localized upon the

---

[4] At first, the heart anlage is a tissue fold that collects intercellular substances. The more the heart grows, the more it is able to carry out rhythmical activity, which leads blood to the brain anlage. This process begins at the fourth week. The bloodstream expands the heart wall. In the expansion (dilation) field, the cells grow into muscle cells.

base of the heart near the aortic outflow and pulmonary outflow (second intercostal spaces, right and left).

The osteopath's left hand lies under the thorax, at the level of the fourth to fifth thoracic vertebrae. It serves as a counterforce for the inductive impulses of the right hand upon the lower sternocostal area. By slight induction to the right or left, the osteopath will screen the capability of the mediastinum to adapt to an impulse. In this way, he or she could estimate if the heart in the pericardial sac is more orientated to the venous return or to the arterial outflow.

The question one should ask is this: Is the heart preferentially organized in a diastolic function or in a systolic function? By delicate and slight inductive maneuvers, the osteopath can create a balance point in the pericardial sac that enables the pericard and the heart to find a better fascial environment in the thorax. Systole and diastole become balanced, and the whole body function becomes better coordinated.

The reason why this happens is simple: By balancing the systolic and diastolic momenta of the heart, the hemodynamic parameters of the whole body become more powerful, and the metabolic fields of the whole body become better irrigated. This results in two remarkable events—the potentializing of the spaces of the body (peritoneal, retroperitoneal, mediastinal, cerebral) and the erection of the body. Instead of being dependent upon hinge points at subsequent levels of the body, the heart can open its own fields of interaction.

6.6 Vasculogenesis as an important informer for heart function

Vasculogenesis seems to be associated with the growth of structures that are in close exchange with the vascular channels. The angioblasts, which function as endothelial cell precursors, constitute the major population of cells participating in the construction of vascular vessels. They arise from most mesodermal tissues of the body except for the prechordal mesoderm. [15] They can migrate,

organize local sprouting, and coalesce in situ to form blood vessels.

It is important to notice that the major source of the vascular endothelium is found in local mesoderm associated with particular developing functions. Most of the angioblasts seem to be associated with splanchnic mesoderm and are intimately related to the metabolic and mechanical changes that are associated with this particular tissue. They react to local environmental cues that determine the morphological pattern of a blood vessel.

Some of the vessels are dependent upon information coming from the neural crest. The large arteries at the outflow tract of the heart are especially organized in synergy with special interference from migrating neural crest cells.

The local mesoderm of organs can be the substrate for vasculogenesis, just as mesenchyme from other tissues can serve as an attractive pole for vascular sprouting. It is certain that organ primordia produce their own attracting factor, and that, through these means, a large part of the organic metabolic content is "translated" to the developing heart. Even the endocardium is informed and formed by angioblastic cells originating in other tissues.

Transition into, and differentiation of, arterial vessels and venous vessels seem to be orchestrated by components of ephrins (EphB2 and EphB4, respectively) and neuregulins (Nrgl1) that serve as transcription factors or signalling molecules. It is remarkable that, at a molecular level, these same transcription factors are the major compounds for differentiation and organization of the primitive brain anlage.

Rather than the blood vessels being considered as outgrowths from the heart, it could be preferable to consider the blood vessels as the main informers of the heart. They transmit not only pressure and volume, but probably also the molecular and metabolic "intimacy" from the various body regions to the center.

The arteries and veins can be studied in their physical parameters, but they should also be considered as a metabolic field participating in the laws of homeostasis of the body. One could even consider the peripheral microcapillary beds as extrapolated microhearts—governed by local metabolic and hemodynamic needs and possessing their own physiology for handling sudden changes in pressure and exchange of metabolites and immune components.

Vascular tonus is not only dependent upon physical cues, but it is certainly co-organized by a delicate balancing between endothelium-derived relaxing factors (EDRF) and endothelium-derived contracting factors (EDCF). The blood vessel can be considered as an endocrinium possessing its own neurovascular tonus and its own endocrinological interactions. According to this view, the laws of Bayliss-Starling and of Laplace seem to be local physical adaptive modalities of the heart upon environmental information, which depends, in turn, upon a tonus organized by distant tissues and organs.

6.7 Conceiving adult heart function and dysfunction

From an embryological viewpoint, one can ascertain that the heart, as an early asymmetrical structure and form, has constructed its function upon the bloodstream entering the porta venosa. The physical laws of pressure and volume that governed this inflow tract made it possible for the heart to express a modified potency of pressure and rhythm, which leaves the heart via the outflow tract (porta arteriosa).

One could ask if it is the blood that "moves" the heart, or if the heart is obliged to transform the energy of the incoming blood into an altered rhythmical pulsating pattern. The heart could be conceived of as one of the first large rhythmic transformers of the body. The metabolic and toxic valences of the digestive and urogenital system are transmitted to the heart by venous pressure and volume, and they are transformed in rhythmic pulsations that are finely attuned in the inotropic, chronotropic, and dromotropic properties of the heart. It is as if the molecular field information is transformed in a subtle rhythmic pulsating field, which must be made accessible for brain interpretation and for supporting a constantly modified consciousness field. By means of the heart, it is possible for the brain to interpret the periphery of the body and to form a better "body chart" of it. The brain transforms the rhythmic impulses of the heart into higher frequency patterns (Hz), which serve consciousness and memory stacking.

The interaction between the blood and the heart can express harmonious patterns of exchange: "the heart can only pump the volume it receives from the periphery." That is the law.

However, it could sometimes be the case that the heart is not able to handle the incoming volume, causing it to make internal adaptations (hypertrophy or dilatation). In other cases, the heart may not possess the needed adaptive capabilities, causing part of the blood volume to be "stocked" in other parts of the body. The venous overflow is mainly handled in the abdominal field, where large quantities of venous blood are stocked in the mesenteric network. The arterial overflow could be aggressive, displaying strong shock waves that destabilize tiny vessels and disturb vital exchange between surfaces, or that create inflammatory episodes that shortcut normal local physiology.

The lungs and their fascial envelopes are especially involved in absorbing an important part of the "small circulation" of the heart. Changes in intrathoracic, intrapleural, and intra-alveolar pressure are logical consequences of the altered state of blood pressure that disturbs normal fascial vitality. In addition, the fasciae and the bones of the cranium possess strong tissue and bony inlets, which are usually organized in a sigmoid form (eg, the canalis carotidis in the temporal bone, the sigmoid sulcus in the cavernous sinus of the sphenoid bone).

The abdomen organizes fascial inlets at the great arterial entrees using the peritoneal passageways, almost like a sphincter. Some organs, such as the spleen, could be conceived of as potential buffers for excess blood volume entering the abdominal cavity. The spleen is quite possibly a masterpiece when it comes to handling the outflowing arterial blood, through its ability to stock it in the multiple splenic sinuses (ie, pulpa rubra splenica). This subtle handling could alter the complete circulating blood volume (eg, hypovolemia).

A change in venous blood volume will probably first be handled in the heart through changing pressure/volume relationships. Another portion of the incoming venous volume is constantly handled by the valveless venous plexuses, which link the spinal venous system to the venous "spare tank" at the base of the brain. This system functions as an overflow system in both directions. If a venous volume presented to the heart is too great, part can be transmitted into this valveless spinal-cerebral venous shunt system. This system can also serve as a fast shunt for balancing the sudden pressure changes that could disturb normal brain compliance.

The excess of systolic volume is handled in an analogous way at the periphery of the heart. First, the volume displacement is slowed down, absorbed, or buffered in some peripheral fascial or visceral spare tanks—that is, organs fitted with a large net of intravisceral sinusoids or a reticular endothelium. By this process, the organs lessen the aggressive influence of the systole upon the subtle exchange areas of the body. Later, the spare tank function of the periphery is able to change central volume handling (ie, activation or inhibition of central baroreceptors by altered renin-angiotensin concentrations).

Another possibility is that the fascia becomes the victim of the pressure and volume overload, resulting in changes to its intrinsic vitality. Subtle changes in osmotic, oncotic, and gaseous pressure may alter the vital equilibrium between acid and alkaline balancing of the intracellular and extracellular environment. This could lead to a state of acidification or alkalinization of the whole body. A global state of acidification apparently activates the ergotropic nuclei of the hypothalamus and organizes a sympathetic tonus of the body. An alkalinized state activates the trophotropic nuclei and organizes a vagal tonus. [16]

It is also known that a continuous degree of acidification of skeletal muscles can progressively interfere with the endocardial/myocardial microvascular beds, leading to "preparation" for coronary suffering. The myofascial system is, in a certain way, determining the metabolic state of the heart muscle and its intima.

The first molecular and cellular adaptations made by the heart primordium around the primary fluid stream are physiological "try outs" for organizing the pressure values of the whole body by means of selecting incoming and outgoing messages. The heart is not only a pump, but also a selective endocrinium that integrates and emits subtle molecular messages. All adaptive behavior of the heart should be conceived of as a fractal-like evolution upon these first subtle impressions.

The heart receives energy from the incoming blood. It transforms the energy into biochemical components in the heart cells by subtle Ca^2 handling and translates those components into mechanical energy, which is reflected in a specific cross-bridging pattern of actin and myosin filaments. [17, 18] And so the cycle perpetuates itself.

The heart possesses three levels of interaction and continuity in its center. Between these three levels, the heart builds lemniscates (energetic continuities) of energy transmission and transformation:

- Blood energy is converted into biochemical energy.
- Biochemical energy is converted into mechanical contractile and propulsive energy.
- Mechanical energy is returned as blood energy.

During its embryological and organogenetic development, the heart develops the possibility of organizing a memory system in its interior. As previously indicated, the continuous and progressive increase of plasma/blood volumes entering the primitive ventricle "sculpts" the heart's interior into a landscape of tiny endothelial cords, called trabeculae (> Fig. 6.5). Each trabecula can be thought of as an expression of

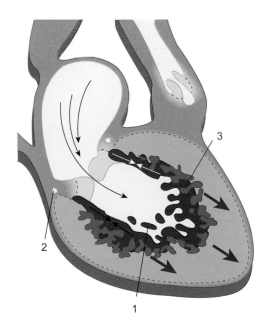

Fig. 6.5 The hemodynamic components of the primitive inflow tract are important in orientating the trabeculae of the heart. Trabeculae create a kind of early memory inside the heart, reflecting the early hemodynamic components that shaped the endocardial landscape.

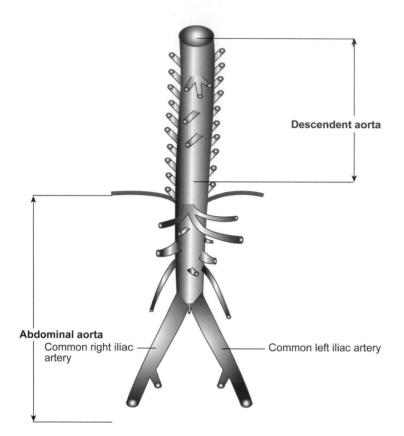

Descendent aorta

Abdominal aorta
Common right iliac
artery

Common left iliac artery

Fig. 6.6 The arterial tree of the body demonstrates the multiplicity of the central branching of the aorta and the complexity of the different hemodynamic components entering and informing the heart.

a particular time/space unit, referring to a certain blood volume entering the heart and sculpting the primitive endothelium. Thus, the story of the entering blood in the heart cavity is laid down as the cartography of the endocard/myocard articulation.

Each time the heart contracts, it gives away a certain unit of power that has already been converted in a spiraling pulse wave. This wave enters one of the main vascular branches of the heart and informs the brain (through the aorta/carotid system) or the lungs (through the pulmonary artery trunk) in its own particular way. These spiraling power units were described by Goncharenko as vortices (or blood spirals) that pass mainly through the cerebral and pulmonary blood beds, transmitting part of the fractal power and memory of the heart to receptive areas in these tissues.

According to this concept, the heart is not only functioning as a pump, but it is becoming one of the main informers of the brain—translating the local stories of the body into energetic values that can

activate and accelerate the responsiveness and alertness of the brain and the lungs. One should remember that each organ has its own receptive microvascular field and its own level of memory stacking. We discuss the brain and the lungs here, because they apparently receive the major trunks of the arterial system of the heart. [19]

The presented figures display the complexity of the cardiac information that circulates to the periphery of the body (➤ Fig. 6.6, ➤ Fig. 6.7).

On a more mechanical-functional level, the heart builds interactions with:
- a neurovascular mesenchyme (base of the heart and the great arteries interact with the peripheral blood vessels)
- its own myofascial environment (pericard and epicard interact with parietal pleura)
- its own biokinetic muscle power (contractility interacts with intracardial volume changes).

In its integration of external and internal forces, the heart expresses a pre-load and after-load force

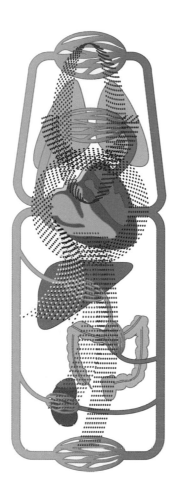

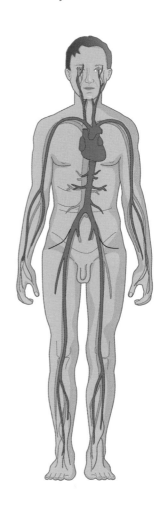

Fig. 6.7 The vascular-interstitial closed circuit (VICC) further demonstrates the multiplicity of the central branching of the aorta and the complexity of the different hemodynamic components entering and informing the heart.

capable of equilibrating resting volume and contractile sarcomere force (depending upon initial resting length). There are two possible results of this adaptive behavior: either the heart succeeds in adapting to the broad array of information, or it has to compensate by eccentric or concentric hypertrophy of its muscle walls. The compensation will eventually fail, manifesting as subtle signs indicative of chronic heart failure (CHF).

Destabilization of the heart function means that volume overload and/or fascial compression forces the heart to be compressed and squeezed in its anatomical environment. The heart rhythm destabilizes when pressure changes or volume changes exceed the normal adaptive capacities of the heart muscle. Some tissue will be irrigated in excess, undergoing excessive pulsation rather than receiving normal impulses for sustaining physiological exchange. Other

tissue will be submitted to vascular spasm, leading to ischemia.

- Excessive arterial pulsation sooner or later creates inflammatory adaptive processes from the aggressed tissues or organs. Even a third or fourth lumbar intervertebral disc can become aggressed by direct contact with the pulsating abdominal aorta.
- Vascular spasm creates a gradual increase in ischemic and/or necrotic aggression of the tissue.

Cardiovascular disease is a progressive evolution from the periphery to the center. The peripheral vessels and tissues first express the centralizing process that will affect the heart in its properties. The more the vascular domain fails to adapt, the more the central part of the circulatory system has to cope with transient changes in blood volumes and in the composition of O_2/CO_2 concentrations. The heart itself can become ischemic and malnourished. It can change its rhythm, fibrillate, and eventually produce embolic clots. Very soon and abruptly, these clots will reach the lungs or the brain, resulting in stroke or death.

Failure of normal heart physiology may be the main predisposing factor for alterations in brain function, through changes in the vascular support of certain brain areas. Any changes in the intrinsic adaptability of the heart for handling the incoming and outgoing bloodstreams will eventually act as disturbing factors that impede brain adaptability. Thus, in almost all cases, heart failure should be interpreted as a predisposing factor for later brain dysfunction.

Deficiency in heart function can be detected long before the CHF or cerebrovascular accident (CVA) has become an irreversible fact. The heart's dysfunction typically displays three stages of progression:

- peripheral inability to adapt to changes in volume and pressure components
- central disturbance resulting in heart ischemic attacks
- cortical shortcut.

The type of tissue that is indicative of progressing cardiovascular disintegration is also threefold:

- Early degenerative processes are expressed by distension and atonia (loss of tonus) of the venous vascular walls (varices). "The venous pulsation could be a transmitted and integrated rhythm transposed by the pulsating maternal blood. It possesses its own contractility in analogy with what is found for the lymph vessels." [19, 20] During embryogenesis and organogenesis, it is the venous system that gives to the heart and the brain. By its continuous pulsations, it drives the morphodynamic mechanisms of both organs. Later, during postnatal life, the venous system receives from the heart by way of the arterial pulsations. One should consider this subtle inversion during the installation of pathology.
- Central failure is reflected in changing patterns of contractility of the heart muscle (eg, ventricular extrasystoles). The heart can be considered as the meeting place between maternal blood flow and fetal blood flow. The rhythm and the mechanical properties it generates are at a balanced equilibrium between the ancestral pulsating force and newly integrated physical forces.

- When the arterial outflow tract fails to adapt, the result could be the final brain dysfunction. Early signs, such as an aortic arch that is unrolled in chest radiographs or respiratory distress syndromes, could be precursors for later brain failure.

The osteopath should be aware of, and remain sensitive to, the progression of these insidious episodes, which focus on a centralized pathology. It is the bloodstream that creates life or shortcuts its own vitality by means of the integrity of its vascular wall. The vascular wall has to be re-evaluated as a complete and independent organ that establishes:

- contractile force (muscle)
- neurovascular reflex activity
- endocrine secretory activity.

The myofascial environment can compress the blood vessels, which then may display deficient vascular tonus by lack of balance in their proper neuroendocrinium (ie, the vascular endothelium and its associated local or distant physiological area). The vessels may also be aggressive for the domain they irrigate or drain through an excess of volume or pulsation. An intelligent brain and intelligent hands should be able to make a distinction between these different possibilities.

Perhaps we need to add an additional principle to that of Dr. Sutherland's thinking, knowing, feeling, and intelligent fingers—namely, that of working with *open hands and an open mind*. This means that the osteopath has to constantly be aware of unforeseen information that is offered by the tissue being studied during synchronization with the body of the patient. The information gathered may not always belong to the symptom being evaluated at that particular moment. Rather, it could belong to well-defined but hidden timescales for which the body tries to compensate by altering its intrinsic physiology.

6.8 The power of blood

Blood is known as a rhythmic fluid able to support metabolic and gaseous exchanges. It orientates different immunological and inflammatory episodes, and it participates in hydrostatic pressure expansion. It can be considered as "motor" and as "constructive" in the interrelation between structure and function. Dr. Sutherland described it as a fluid mesoderm, a flowing intermediate, pulsating upon the tides of the heart, the brain, and all other metabolic fields, and supporting the final homeostatic valences of the body.

The embryological record indicates that there is a blood circulation without heart function in the early stages of development. Blood apparently does not need a "motor." Rather, it seems to be able to function upon intrinsic physical parameters.

One could ascertain that the primordium of the heart is formed by the early blood dynamics. As we have previously indicated, the blood, as a vitalizing tool, displays different functional sequences. They can be conceived of as periods of importance in constructing the metabolic fields of the different germ layers.

The venous bloodstream organized initially by the umbilical vesicle and later by the placental vascular bed, is converted progressively into an arterial vascular bed at the inside of the embryo. The heart is progressively formed as a pulsating answer upon the intrinsically pulsating and rhythmic properties of the ancestral venous blood and upon the steadily increasing peripheral resistances of the fields it has to irrigate.

We previously mentioned that the primitive endothelium of the heart tube functions as an early metabolic field in which the pulsations of the venous inflow carve the historical cartography of embryonic circulation into a dynamic pattern represented by the heart trabeculae. Dependent upon the physiological parameters of preload and afterload, the heart will use these microtimes of endocardial impressions as fluctuating "hinge points" for affording appropriate information to the brain and periphery. One has to emphasize that the brain is an intimate part of the body—not a separate, specialized unit governing all the laws of life.

- The vitelline and umbilical bloodstreams consolidate the first pathways by which the venous blood creates the substrate (material components) for organ construction and emplacement. Blechschmidt described them as the "permeation" and "permeation" fluxes of the gastrula and the early embryonic body.

- The arterial blood creates the orientation of each organ by dynamic patterns of increasing blood pressure, volume changes, and rhythmic pulsation.
- The venous-arteriolar interweaving can be considered as a privileged metabolic field in which metabolic activity is supported by the physical values of the pulsating blood. The blood pressure and volume create a "blood lake" in which all necessary information can be expressed.
- The venous return to the heart informs the latter about the metabolic and peripheral sequences that occurred, such as volume changes and metabolic exchanges (eg, toxicity, metabolic waste).
- The heart itself is built in the same manner as the peripheral blood beds. A web of hairpin vessels and blood lakes, which initially slow the circulating blood, forms this organ. The heart accumulates blood from the periphery into a functional center and creates a contractile force through volume expansion and elastic recoil.

One can conclude that the organs of the body organize a network for the bloodstream, and the heart creates a rhythm for blood pulsation dependent upon peripheral resistance. By the third month of embryological development, one can find an integrated venous network.

6.8.1 The basics of the venous bloodstream anlage

An important developmental sequence is that the embryonic bloodstream progressively changes from a paired anlage to an asymmetrical pattern orientated by the incoming venous vessels. Before closure, one can already find an asymmetrical pattern in the venous system that is in direct contact with the neural tube. The vena umbilicalis sinistra (left umbilical vein) seems more powerful than the right umbilical vein, indicating the first signs of asymmetry in the embryo. This fact can be verified at stage 9 in the human embryo (26 days postfertilization), as depicted by O'Rahilly.

The venous income directs the early bloodstream into a right-shift organization, first in the peritoneal area and later in the pleuropericardial cavity. The anatomical substrate of this right-shift is the construction of the vena cava and vena porta. This right-shift is not a consequence of the rotation of the intestine, but rather an independent intrinsic pattern of the venous blood stream. It could be created by subtle metabolic exchanges between the early placenta anlage and the early organ anlage. The major organs integrating this right-shift impulse are the duodenum loop and the liver bud.

6.8.2 The basics of the arterial pulsating field[5]

- The basic arterial system is symmetrically organized at the beginning of embryonic development.
- The paired aorta anlage is a plexus of hairpin vessels. During the fourth week, there is a development toward a single configuration—the basic dorsal aorta. The paired original organization can be found in the cephalad (neck region) and caudal (umbilical region) positions.
- During the ninth week, the aorta migrates slightly to the left of the vertebral column.
  This migration is due to the early twisting of the aorta during maturation of the conotruncus of the heart. The main arterial blood flows toward the head, and the trunk becomes left orientated.
- Collaterals of the aorta are built during the construction of the metameric and visceral compartments.

The aortic arch system is dependent upon the branchial arch construction. The branchial arches help to construct an *indirect* arterial pathway toward the right side of the brain by the brachiocephalic trunk, as well as a *direct* relation between the heart and the brain over the aortic arch and common carotid artery. The left carotid artery and the left brachiocephalic vessels are in direct functional and anatomical continuity with left ventricle activity, and they probably express a different arterial peak flow than that of the right arterial branching to the head.

This asymmetric arterial flow could be an important morphogenetic factor in informing the right and left sides of the brain differently during embryogenesis. Studying the arterial impulse and impact upon the embryonic brain allows one to establish a continuous deflection of the anterior telencephalic/mesencephalic unit upon the posterior rhombencephalic unit during the vascular cardiac impulse[6].

- The aortic arch not only builds the mechanical equilibrium point for right arm growth expansion, but it also constructs a direct passageway for the rhythmic activity of the left arm. Force and power (right arm orientation) are linked by the aortic arch to subtlety and handiness (left arm orientation).
- The left carotid receives a direct, powerful impulse from the heart, orientating the hydrostatic pressure to the brain area. One might suppose that the left side will experience abrupt changes in pressure and rhythm of heart activity more intensely than the right side. However, the mechanical power of the heart is deviated in a large siphoning system at the inside of the skull (circle of Willis, arterial flexures in the petrous bone and cavernous sinus).

Nevertheless, the arterial impulse might be so powerful that it could be capable of orientating the skull and the cortex in a left backward spiral rotation pattern. This hypothesis is supported by the fact that, starting at three-and-a-half weeks postfertilization, the motion of the heart already expresses a detectable mechanical input upon the brain. [19]

One can imagine this left backward spiraling by looking up toward the left with the left eye, and rotating and extending the head toward the left. It is evident to suppose that brain activity could be largely supported by this incoming left spiraling arterial bloodstream.

The venous blood of the head and left arm is concentrated in the left innominate vein, flowing to the right heart. This indicates a right downward spiraling into the vena cava superior. One can imagine this right forward and downward spiraling when one looks downward and to the right foot with the left eye.

---

[5] O'Rahilly R, Müller F. The Embryonic Human Brain: An Atlas of Developmental Stages. Hoboken, NJ: Wiley-Liss, 2006.

[6] King AB, et al. Human forebrain activation by visceral stimuli. *J Comp Neurol.* 1999;413(4):572-582.

6.8.3 Disturbances in bloodstream and fascial organization

These observations should not be interpreted as anatomical or physiological facts. Rather, they are presented as suggestions for the osteopath, to relate his or her findings to functional patterns that could express underlying disturbances in bloodstreams and their related fascial organization. It seems evident to suppose that these main vascular beds are embedded in, and sustained by, major fascial pathways. The lungs counterbalance the right shift system (venous return) by creating a bypass system in the heart to the left (ductus Botalli, or ductus arteriosus) at about the same time during fetal development.

For this chapter, we can conclude that the heart itself is a transformed organ depending upon the continuously changing mechanical and metabolic impulses of the incoming and outgoing bloodstream. The bloodstream transmits the peripheral needs and resistances to this fluidic force plate in order to accommodate normal physiology.

During early embryonic evolution, the heart represents nothing more than an answer to the periphery. It continues to do so during adult life by adapting its inner physiology to pressure and volume changes expressed by preload and postload values.

A more subtle vision about the left- and right-shifts of the vascular beds of the heart could be as follows: They contribute to the capacities of the individual to adapt intelligent needs to a changing environment. [21]

6.9 The heart and the brain

Is the cerebrospinal fluid (CSF) flow an independent dynamic flow, or is it vitalized by the heart pulsation? In this section, we will consider whether the CSF displays dynamic properties by intrinsic force, or whether this fluid is pulsed by external forces that interfere with the anatomical environment in which it is produced. The heart and the pulsation of blood could be conceived of as important factors in determining force, velocity, and electromagnetic equilibrium of the CSF flow.

It may be appropriate here to provide a brief review of the scientific observations concerning the production and flow of the CSF.

Medical imaging has made much progress during the past few decades. It is by this means that greater understanding has been obtained about the flow of the CSF. Computed tomography- (CT-) ventriculography and magnetic resonance imaging (MRI) have revealed specific patterns of flow of this "precious fluid." [22, 23]

The dynamics of the CSF have been studied mostly from a pathological perspective. Most of these studies have been aimed at diagnosing or finding etiologic factors that induce specific patterns of hydrocephalus. [24] Indirectly, the importance of a non-obstructed CSF flow for the maintenance of brain function and the equilibrium of biochemical imaging of the brain and brain fluids was discovered and updated.

The passage of the CSF into the subarachnoideal spaces and from there into the subarachnoideal villi and veins seems necessary to eliminate waste products from the cortical areas. This fluid pressure also assures the mechanical protection of the brain. By studying the dynamics of the CSF, one discovers the importance of its biochemical and electromagnetic equilibrium in maintaining normal vitality of the corticomedullar unit and the peripheral nerve trajectories.

Several biological facts may be useful to review.

The typical adult possesses about 135 mL of CSF inside the cerebrospinal fluctuation, though only about 35 mL circulate inside the ventricles. These values vary slightly between males and females. The reason for a greater circulating CSF volume in males might be related to the typically greater cranial volume of men. In addition, an increase in CSF volume can apparently be established in old age, especially in males. However, one should note that there does not exist any difference between the intraventricular volumes in males and females. [25]

The biochemical constitution of the CSF resembles the ultrafiltrate of the blood. The first step in the formation of this fluid is the passage of the ultrafiltrate of the plasma across the "nontight-junctions" of choroid capillaries at the level of the choroid villus. Another part of the fluid could be produced by the cells of the tela ependymalis lining the ventricles. This ultrafiltration happens through changes in hydrostatic pressure variations in the choroid plexuses and by active secretion at the level of the ependymal cells.

One should note that recent research underlines the importance of the cerebral parenchyma in producing a major part of the CSF. [26] The parenchyma could represent an important surface for fluctuant (phasic) secretion and absorption of CSF via paravascular pathways—without participation of the formerly described and studied pathways for secretion and absorption.

Next, the ultrafiltrate is transformed into the CSF secretion by means of active metabolic processes inside the choroid epithelium. [22, 24] This production of CSF happens at the choroid plexuses of all the different ventricles, as well as at the level of the ventricular ependymal tissue. The choroid plexus at the fourth ventricle might produce more CSF than the plexuses of the lateral ventricles. The production of this fluid happens at a rate of 0.4 mL/min.

A flux of CSF displacement is created between the areas of production and absorption. The normal pattern is a displacement of the flux via the ventricles, first toward the subarachnoideal space and next toward the subarachnoideal villi. The absorption finishes when the fluid is integrated into the sagittal veins inside the dural membranes. [23, 27]

The following trajectory was described during an MRI study:

- The CSF flows out from the lateral ventricles through the two foramina of Monro (interventricular foramina) and into the third ventricle. Then it flows caudally across the aqueductus Sylvii into the fourth ventricle.
- Passing through the foramina of Luschka, the main portion of CSF goes to the cisterna pontocerebellaris and to the cisterna pontis.
- The largest flow of CSF is received by the foramen of Magendie, which dispatches the fluid to all the remaining subarachnoideal spaces, most importantly the cisterna basalis.

The absorption, as previously mentioned, happens at the level of the Pacchionian villi, though these projections are most important in quick absorption of the CSF during rapid intracranial pressure expansion. Other portions of CSF are exchanged at the level of the Virchow-Robin space or drained by the principal spinal and cranial nerves. Still another portion is drained in the circumventricular organs (ie, subfornical organ, pineal body, pituitary gland, area postrema, and choroid plexus). [28, 29]

The flow of CSF is not a rectilinear trajectory. Rather, an alternating forward-backward movement can be observed during the fluid's final propulsion toward the foramen of Magendie. Du Boulay [30] calculated that, during a normal heart rhythm of 70 to 80 beats/min, a volume of 7 to 8 mL of CSF is displaced inside the third ventricle. This forward-backward movement is responsible for creating turbulence phenomena at the foramina of Monro, especially at the level of the Sylvian aqueduct.

Physical/mechanical parameters, such as sudden changes in diameter, could be responsible for these phenomena. [31] Nevertheless, identical turbulence phenomena have been established at the floor of the fourth ventricle. A higher velocity has been found at the ventricle floor, as opposed to the ventricle corpus, where the stream velocity was found to be lesser. The passage of CSF in the aqueduct of Sylvius finally displays a velocity of 4 to 6 cm/sec.

Apparently, a number of different factors are responsible for the propulsion of CSF:

- The continuous formation of CSF.
- Ventricular pulsation related to arterial pulsation.
- Ciliary action of the ventricular ependymal layer.
- Pressure gradients at the level of the arachnoideal villi.
- Factors 1 and 4 are also mentioned by J. Upledger [32] as important elements to explain the biphasic character of the cranial rhythmic impulse (CRI).))
- Factor 2 is quite an)interesting and attractive assessment. H.I. Magoun, in his book, *Osteopathy in the Cranial Field,* stated that the electrical activity of the cortex, the activity of the glial cells, and the pulsation of the CSF collaborate to determine the final expression of the CRI.
- Factor 3 has been interpreted by Upledger and Magoun differently:)
  – According to Upledger, the ependymal layer is a specific place for proprioceptive feedback out of the sutures of the cranium (which can be distended by increasing or decreasing intracranial pressure).
  – According to Magoun, the ependymal cells belong to the activating mechanism of CSF flow, together with the glial cells.

Ventricular pulsation seems to be supported by external factors that depend mainly on the pulsating force of the bloodstream.

- Du Boulay, who was previously mentioned, observed rhythmic pump activity of the third ventricle at the moment that both thalamic nuclei were squeezed by the systolic brain expansion.
- The PRIMIS [23] group at the University of Brussels developed two different image displays of CSF flow, during systolic and diastolic heart dynamics.
- The work of P.C. Njemanze and O.J. Beck [33] points in the same direction. They established a more pronounced CSF flow during heart systole, compared to diastole.

The increase of flow has been assessed in the fourth ventricle, the foramen of Magendie, the cisterna magna, and the cervical and spinal subarachnoideal spaces. The foramina of Monro dilate during systole and retract during diastole; the same is evident for the aqueduct of Sylvius. The third ventricle displays an increase in height during systole, and a decrease during diastole.

Interesting for osteopathy in the cranial field is the relation of the dynamics of CSF flow to the integrity of the cardiovascular system. This "third circulation," as defined by the CSF flow, is largely associated with the dynamics of the heart and the blood power.

By studying the embryological steps of brain development, one is reminded that the brain begins its specific activity only at the moment that it is "invaded" by mesenchymal cells, which accompany sufficient blood supply to the brain. A logical hypothesis could be that both the activity of the brain and the quality of its CRI are sustained by an intact cardiovascular system. This further implies that cardiovascular symptomatology—or even such precursor signs as simple venous stasis (eg, hepatojugular hyperpressure)—could be a subtle indicator of a beginning cerebrospinal deterioration.

The question remains: Is the CSF flow an intrinsic dynamic fact, or is it activated by the power of blood?

A more historical dilemma appears when we study two statements, of Still and Sutherland:

- "The role of the artery is supreme."
- "The CSF is on command."

We now know that the CSF serves as a buffer fluid to accommodate sudden increases in intracranial venous pressure due to intrathecal obstacles or due to arterial/venous deficient exchange (➤ Fig. 6.8, ➤ Fig. 6.9). This function of pressure absorption and diffusion by the CSF compartments largely supports the physiological integrity of the brain and is a determinant cofactor of brain compliance. The CSF functions as a fluid that can rapidly be drained into the cisterns of the brain or into the spinal arachnoideal compartment. By that means, it supports the compliance capacity of the brain by preventing excessive intrathecal pressure and subsequent ischemic damage.

The brain needs this "waterjacket" as an ambient milieu for conserving its functional integrity. When pressure becomes too high, it will be compressed, and ischemia of certain brain areas will appear. When pressure is too low, the brain fields become

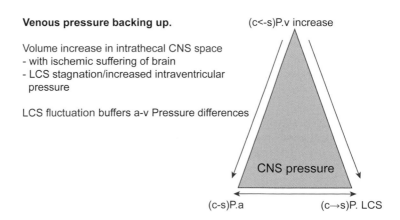

Fig. 6.8 A diagram of compliance regulation of the brain indicates the different components regulating CNS and intrathecal pressure. Much of the fluid balance of the brain is dependent upon how venous pressure can be accommodated by the cavities surrounding the brain and by the ways venous blood pressure is buffered by the dynamic components of CSF flow.

Venous pressure backing up.

Volume increase in intrathecal CNS space
- with ischemic suffering of brain
- LCS stagnation/increased intraventricular
  pressure

LCS fluctuation buffers a-v Pressure differences

(c<-s)P.v increase

CNS pressure

(c-s)P.a   (c→s)P. LCS

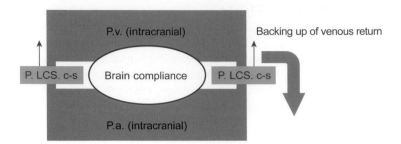

Fig. 6.9 A diagram of cranial intrathecal pressure regulation further indicates the different components regulating CNS and intrathecal pressure. Much of the fluid balance of the brain is dependent upon how venous pressure can be accommodated by the cavities surrounding the brain and by the ways venous blood pressure is buffered by the dynamic components of CSF flow.

"dry," and the brain will increasingly need to find support upon nuclei and other cerebral structures to guarantee its function.

It is clear that not all developmental hinge points (eg, flexures, NEP fields [34]) of the brain that are used during its embryological development continue to serve as mechanical references for brain enfolding and positioning. Instead, they are transformed into integrative centers serving cognition and autonomic function. Thus, when the brain is no longer capable of "swimming" in its waterjacket, it needs to find supplementary support upon loci that do not serve this purpose. Nuclei and commissures may become compressed and express either an exaggerated or inhibited pattern. Normal motion and position of the amygdala, for example, could be impaired, leading to the eliciting of a compulsive or obsessive behavior, such as fear, anxiety, or aggression.

An osteopath who understands the laws of mechanical and fluid exchange of the brain with its environment will certainly be capable of helping this structure, by reassuring normal intracranial and intrathecal pressure gradients. It is evident, of course, that not all psychological and psychiatric disorders can be reduced to an impaired fluid exchange of the brain. Therefore, it is important to underline that a multidisciplinary approach is usually the most appropriate way of interfering with the brain problem. In any case, it should be clear to the osteopath that the brain is not a separate, independent part of the body. Rather, it is fully integrated with the rest of the body, and its autonomy is dependent upon all the valences worked out by the body.

The brain uses all the microtimes of its development for forming a landscape of the body that can be used as both an integrative tool and a source of information for the body about its own functioning or other conceptual purposes. These two uses are logical expressions of the embryological and organogenetic maturation of brain function and structure, which reflects a bottom-up patterning for the immature brain and a top-down patterning during adult life. The brain employs this body landscape as a feedback mechanism for reinforcing or inhibiting the physiology of the whole system. In that way, the brain is dependent upon all the fields from which it gathers information (eg, metabolic, rhythmic, urogenital).

The blood has the power of informing the brain by means of physical values transformed in rhythmic impulses, flow patterns, and vortices, which can alter the statics, dynamics, and intrinsic rhythms of the brain.

REFERENCES
[1] Carlson MB. Human Embryology and Developmental Biology. St. Louis, MO: Mosby-Year Book, 1994:372.
[2] O'Rahilly R, Müller F. The early development of the hypoglossal nerve and occipital somites in staged human embryos. Am J Anat. 1984;169(3):237–257.
[3] Stelzner F. Die chirurgische Anatomie der Grenzlamellen der Schilddrüse und die Nervi laryngei. Langenbecks Arch Chir. 1988;373(6):355–366.
[4] Debrunner W. Struktur und Funktion des menschlichen Herzbeutels. Z Anat Entwicklungsgesch. 1956;119(6):512–537.
[5] Carlson MB. Human Embryology and Developmental Biology. St. Louis, MO: Mosby- Year Book, 1994:411.

[6] Myers MM, et al. Relationships between breathing activity and heart rate in fetal baboons. Am J Physiol. 1990;258(6 Pt 2):R1479–1485.

[7] Chairopoulos P. Les poumons prennent de l'air. Science et vie. 1995:98–106.

[8] Trudinger BJ, Cook CM. Fetal breathing movements. Early Hum Dev. 1989;20:247–253.

[9] Hinrischsen KV. Human Embryologie. Heidelberg, Germany: Springer Verlag, 1990:221–222.

[10] De la Cruz MV, Markwald RR, eds. Living Morphogenesis of the Heart. Boston, MA: Birkäuser, 1998.

[11] Manasek FJ, Monroe RG. Early cardiac morphogenesis is independent of function. Dev Biol. 1972;27(4):584–588.

[12] Steding G, Seidl W. Contribution to the development of the heart. Part 1: normal development. Thorac Cardiovasc Surg. 1980;28(6):386–409.

[13] Lee JM, Boughner DR. Mechanical properties of human pericardium. Differences in viscoelastic response when compared with canine pericardium. Circ Res. 1985;57(3):475–481.

[14] Blechschmidt E. Sein und Werden. Stuttgart, Germany: Urachhaus Verlag, 1982:48.

[15] Carlson MB. Human Embryology and Developmental Biology. St. Louis, MO: Mosby-Year Book, 1994:375.

[16] Lamers HJ. Het grondsysteem volgens Pischinger. Congres on neuraltherapie; 1985.

[17] Lakatta EG. Functional implications of spontaneous sarcoplacmic reticulum Ca2++ release in the heart. Cardiovasc Res. 1992;26(3):193–214.

[18] Priebe H-J, Skarvan K. Cardiovascular Physiology. London, United Kingdom: BMJ Publishing Group, 1995:25–61.

[19] O'Rahilly R, Müller F. The Embryonic Human Brain: An Atlas of Developmental Stages. Hoboken, NJ: Wiley & Sons, 2006.

[20] Degenhardt BP, Kuchera ML. Update on osteopathic medical concepts and the lymphatic system. J Am Osteopath Assoc. 1996;96(2):97–100.

[21] Wilmar F. Vorgebürtliche Menschwerdung. Stuttgart, Germany: Mellinger Verlag, 1991:92–120.

[22] Zentner J, et al. CT-ventriculography to control the passage of cerebrospinal fluid. Technical note. Acta Neurochir. 1987;89(3-4):140–143.

[23] PRIMIS group. Dynamische beelden van de beweging van het hersenvocht by de mens via MRB. Vrije Universiteit Brussel (VUB) magazine. 1988.

[24] Wocjan J, et al. Analysis of CSF dynamics by computerized pressure-elastance resorption test in hydrocephalic children. Childs Nerv Syst. 1986;2(2):98–100.

[25] Grant R, et al. Human cranial CSF volumes measured by MRI: sex and age influences. Magn Reson Imaging. 1987;5(6):465–468.

[26] Iliff JJ, et al. A paravascular pathway facilitates CSF flow through the brain parenchyma and the clearance of interstitial solutes, including amyloid β. Sci Transl Med. 2012;4(147):147ra111.

[27] Breeze RE, et al. CSF production in acute ventriculitis. J Neurosurg. 1989;70(4):619–622.

[28] Feinberg DA, Mark AS. Human brain motion and cerebrospinal fluid circulation demonstrated with MR velocity imaging. Radiology. 1987;163(3):793–799.

[29] Hashimoto PH. Aspects of normal cerebrospinal fluid circulation and circumventricular organs. Prog Brain Res. 1992;91:439–443.

[30] Sherman JL, Citrin CM. Magnetic resonance demonstration of normal CSF flow. AJNR Am J Neuroradiol. 1986;7(1):3–6.

[31] Malko JA, et al. A phantom study of intracranial CSF signal loss due to pulsatile motion. AJNR Am J Neuroradiol. 1988;9(1):83–89.

[32] Upledger JE, Vredevoogd JD. Craniosacral Therapy. Vista, CA: Eastland Press, 1983.

[33] Njemanze PC, Beck OJ. MR-gated intracranial CSF dynamics: evaluation of CSF pulsatile flow. AJNR Am J Neuroradiol. 1989;10(1):77–80.

[34] Bayer SA, Altman J. The Human Brain During the Early First Trimester. Boca Raton, FL: CRC Press, 2008.

6

CHAPTER 7

The fascial concept and its history in osteopathic philosophy

7.1 Introduction

By considering the evolution of the fascial concept throughout osteopathic history, we notice that the fascia has been increasingly studied as a well-established organ. The notion of "linking tissue" without any vital interference on the biochemical and biophysical level has gradually disappeared.

Although A.T. Still mentioned all the possible faculties of the fascia, it took a long time before this tissue's biochemical and biophysical properties became sufficiently elucidated and applicable in the manual approach of the patient. Yet even now, the predominant opinion about the function of the fascia is that it reacts mechanically upon stretch, and that it is the go-between for muscle and joint. However, in a more advanced opinion, fascia is considered to be a linking tissue or ligamentous organization between different visceral compartments and the parietal sphere.

Furthermore, old definitions of fascia, such as it being a membranous aponeurosis that envelops muscle and covers anatomical regions, remain the most accepted assumptions of traditional medicine. Even the osteopathic language mentions only the first three subdivisions of the connective tissue as belonging to the fascial level—the loose connective tissue, the semi-modeled tissue, and the modeled connective tissue.

According to a more advanced model, however, all connective tissue formations, including the mechanical arranged layers, are capable of expressing cellular and tissue exchanges that influence the homeostasis of the body in an immediate way. Still states this concept as follows:

"Knowledge of the universal extent of the fascia is imperative, and is one of the greatest aids to the person who seeks the causes of disease. It has a network of nerves, cells, and tubes running to and from it; it is crossed and no doubt filled with millions of nerve centers and fibers, which carry on the work of secreting and excreting fluids vital and destructive. By its action we live and by its failure we die." [1]

What can we do today to add to this concept? We can try to explain every part of these ideas with modern medical terminology and knowledge.

Histologically, the fascia should be defined as an unorganized connecting tissue between all distinct levels of bodily functions. It links the mechanical units of the body to the internal fasciae of the body (viscera and central nervous system [CNS]), and it also links the different compartments of these deep fasciae to the axial fascia and the subcutaneous, pannicular fasciae (➤ Fig. 7.1).

Its precursor can be found in the embryonic mesenchyme, which can be considered as the first primitive fascial landscape of the developing body. The balance between embryonic tissue and structure is organized by mesenchymal tissue, itself dependent upon epithelio-mesenchymal transitions (EMT) related to local and structural inductions or interactions of the endodermal and ectodermal layers of the embryo. That means that each part of mesenchymal transformation withholds a particular space/time unit that is organized by a specific mesodermal response. This response, in turn, relies upon fibroblast activation/inhibition or upon activation of neural crest cells (➤ Fig 7.2).

The most important feature for understanding fascia is that it is a linking tissue that is capable of responding with every stretch in any direction without being torn or disrupted. Organized tissues, such as tendons and aponeuroses, respond only upon stretch in a single direction, or else they loose their fibrillous pattern and are destroyed.[1]

The most striking feature about the inner fasciae is that they express an almost complete continuity

---

[1] Willard F. Conference on fasciae at Sutherland Cranial Academy of Belgium; 2012; Louvain-la-Neuve, Belgium.

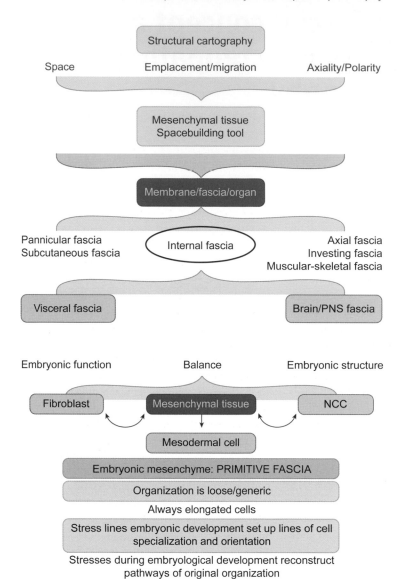

Fig. 7.1 A diagrammatic representation of development from cells to tissue structure reveals that the CNS and visceral compartments of the body are covered by the internal fasciae.

Fig. 7.2 Mesenchyme is the intermediate, balancing structure that supports mechanical and informative function in the embryo.

from their lower level of origin to their final point of insertion. They form a kind of continuous sac that envelops **either** the complete visceral sphere or the complete CNS. This fact confirms the opinion of E. Blechschmidt that, during its development, the nervous system is "gliding" upon the visceral counterpart by means of its fascial construction and reaction pattern, organized by the subarachnoidal space (ascensus cerebri/descensus viscerum).

7.2 Osteopathic concepts integrating the fascia as a tool

7.2.1 A renewed mechanical concept

It was quite a revolution for the pure mechanistic osteopathic concept, which conceived of fascia only as a biomechanical lever of force transmission, when Barral [2] described particular visceral anatomical areas as being "articulated" by fasciae. With this description, he shifted the biomechanical concept to the visceral area and attributed a physiological role to this living tissue. The fascia, as a concept, started to live and to contribute to life.

In addition, Roques and Gabarel [3] talked about "points de rencontre,"[2] indicating that at specific anatomical levels—osseous or ligamentous—fascial sheets interdigitate and build subtle transitions of force-distributing levers. The meaning of their thesis was that the fascia is capable of transmitting subtle tensions from one anatomical area to another without being involved in the specific physiology of this particular area.

Disturbances in the physiology of a maxillary sinus can be transmitted as tensions to a temporal bone by way of the common insertions of the temporal fascial sleeve and the superficial fascia of the face covering the zygomatic bone. In this way, the zygomatic bone becomes the point de rencontre, or force plate, between the two separated areas of the temporal bone and the maxillary sinus. Thus, we now can accept that fasciae articulate osseous, musculoligamentous, and visceral areas. The precise ways in which they exert their integrating, informing, and transmitting tasks will be examined later in this text.
- *A fluidic concept.*
It is widely known that the fascia contains a rich network of vascular and lymphatic terminals that permit arterial-venous and venous-lymphatic exchange. The role it plays in equilibrating the amount of extracellular fluid (ECF) is best understood when we study the vast network of lymphatic lacunae dispersed even in the finest membranes and endothelial organizations of its anatomy.

We can state that the fascia is the organizer of physiological relations between the spared (or stocked) fluids and the circulating body fluids. In a sense, the fascia is like a spare tank for colloids and fluids.

D. Bois [4] states that the triad fascia/blood/lymph manifests itself as a strong organizer of pathology. The fascia and the blood are submitted to particular kinds of trauma, and they integrate physical trauma by osteoarticular or myofascial strains.

They interfere with physical, psychological, and mental stress, and they create psychosomatic tension that alters the total body scheme.

7.2.2 A fluidic cranial concept

Craniosacral therapists agree with the statement that the cerebrospinal fluid (CSF) interferes with the outermost parts of the whole body. The exchange between the CSF and the fasciae takes place over minute liquid propagation through the sheets of the collagen fibers constituting the envelopes of the conducting nerves. This thesis underlines the controlling function of brain homeostasis upon the rest of the body's physiology. Expansion and retraction of the CSF in the brain and medulla can be perceived as flexion-extension or external-internal rotation phases throughout the whole body by means of these tubular connections.

Not only do the neurons contribute to such exchange, but all the fasciae that envelop the brain and medulla could support this rhythmical propagation from the center to the periphery. This statement may seem to be partly contradicted by the fact that most cranial osteopaths interpret disturbances in the craniosacral rhythm as being dependent upon peripheral perturbations originating by visceral or parietal malfunctioning. Therefore, it could also be possible that the craniosacral rhythm expresses a mean value of all the rhythms from all over the body, rather than being a completely independent value. Perhaps when this mean value is ideal (homeostatic), that is the time when the fluctuations in the CSF display a "normal" rhythm of 8 to 14 cycles/minute.

In examining embryological developmental phases of the cortex, one can notice that the brain is the ultimate organ in the development of the embryo. Liver development and heart maturation all serve to distribute the vital fluids into the brain. It should be no wonder that the different qualitative and quantitative fluid oscillations to which the brain is submitted all are integrated in its own pattern. In other words, the brain synthesizes a mean rhythm that expresses an integrated physiology. This hypothesis can be easily defended if one knows that the CSF secretion is dependent upon subtle interactions between the glial cells, which constitute the walls of the

---

[2] point de rencontre = encounter place

brain ventricles, and the choroid plexuses, which protrude into the walls of the ventricles (as roof laminae).

A large portion of brain information is dependent upon the specific moment at which peripheral vascular information intrudes into the early ectoderm formations, supplying the first mesenchymal information to the microglial cells. By studying the embryological development of the brain, we can ascertain that before functioning as a control center, the cortex functions as a large "metabolic field" consuming a great deal of energy. This field is dependent upon peripheral nourishing fluxes that display independent rhythms and wave expansions. The cortex is the main consumer of energy during the entire embryological and fetal history of the body.

The liver and the heart can be thought of as the "servants" of the neuroectodermal Gestaltung. These organs increasingly become the informers of the brain through modifications of metabolic compounds and modifications of rhythm and pulsation. The liver and heart constantly deliver information by means of mechanical bits of the hemodynamic/metabolic fields that support the electrical and neuroendocrine functions of the developing brain. This information is converted by the developing brain into microtimes of cognitive function and memory stacking. In summary, the brain not only builds memory by its own properties of memory stacking, but it receives part of its memory from the liver and heart.

7.2.3 The fascia conceived as a physiological unit

The ECM displays two particularities: it can remain silent for a long time, or it can suddenly be a source of a paroxysm. Silence does not mean that it does not function; it means only that connective tissues, included fasciae, possess a great capacity for integrating and stocking information. The ECM probably takes part in the function of "subconscious" memory of the whole body plan.

Different constituent parts of the connective tissue display their own ways of memory accumulation.

- Collagen fibers are constantly reorganized and restructured according to the mechanical stimuli they experience. The fibrocyte plays an important role in this process, because it is continuously "sensing" its immediate environment by absorbing free amino acids out of the colloidal milieu of the ECM. These amino acids are reorganized into new tropocollagen fibrils in the endoplasmic reticulum and later secreted again into the interstitial fluid as new components of the collagen fibers. [5] This process is similar to early embryonic maturation processes, in which the amniotic fluid is ingested to serve as a nourishing and informing liquid. This fluid stimulates the taste papillae of the tongue. It also fills the bronchial alveolar sprouts with liquid and organizes sufficient hydrostatic pressure to permit further spatial organization of the bronchial tree.

- The amniotic fluid stimulates maturation of the endoluminal surface of the primitive gut. It is excreted with the pro-urine, and the fetus, who is sensing his or her external milieu, "drinks" it. *The fibrocyte is a kind of miniature embryological manufacturer, constantly modifying the inner milieu by changing information arising from the ECM.*

- Properly speaking, the embryo and the fetus are bathed in a liquid, the amniotic fluid, that is filled with polymers, while their genetic code is beginning to be expressed.

- Biochemical information is constantly compared with the genetic program of the cell. The information is integrated or refused as a component of the basic program of DNA, in the form of the four nucleotide bases adenine, cytosine, thymine, and guanine (A, C, T, G). These four bases combine together in groups of three (called triplets, or codons) to form the 20 standard amino acids used by cells to build proteins. There are actually a total of 64 possible combinations of base codons, but some amino acids can be encoded by more than one codon.

- Even if these 64 combinations create an enormous codon chart, still greater combination charts of stored memory are possible. For example, the sugar polymers in the body can be combined into 35,560 possibilities of stored information. This means that these sugar polymers are probably the most accurate and fastest engrammas that can be used by the body to stock urgent information. They could be conceived of as "fieldworkers" functioning under an administrative staff (ie, the genetic codons).

- Another interesting kind of memory is expressed by the immune system, which displays humoral and cellular memory faculties.
- Different kinds of immune reactions can impede normal physiology. Most importantly, the circulating immune complexes can organize major inflammatory and destructive processes at some distance from the original aggression or aggressor. In addition, the allergic, histamine-dependent reactions (eg, IgE stimulation) can immobilize complete anatomical areas.
A more subtle way of inhibiting physiology is carried out by so-called *lymphoplasmatic infiltrates,* which inhibit normal depolarization of cell areas adjacent to the infiltrate. The cells stay depolarized (or hyperpolarized), manifesting as a slowly dying process. Pischinger [6] mentioned these inhibitions as a major source of impediment for body homeostasis.
- Additional, less well-defined manifestations of memory stocking include *the energy cysts* described by Upledger. [7] These cysts display tissue immobility by excessive energy concentration in a particular anatomical area. This concentration of energy organizes itself by an obstruction of the effective electrical conduction capability of the tissue. The energy concentration is defined as an area or a physical state in which the body seems unable to dissipate this concentrated energy as heat or other forms of entropy. On palpation, this tissue appears thickened, congested, and stiffer than normal tissue. It belongs, in most cases, to a well-defined area of the body in which the initial trauma was inserted. Metameric repartition is common for this kind of energy accumulation.

7.2.4 The fascia as a rhythmical tissue

The most evident manifestation of life for humans and other animal species is the capability of mobility. Movement seems to be the most qualified parameter of freedom and is defined in all of its parts by physical parameters. Subjectively, it is lived as a

qualium—a qualitative expression of personal well-being. It is a macroscopic and microscopic observable expedient for exchange with the direct environment.

However, when one considers exchange and environment, one also has to study resistance. The interaction between movement and resistance is perhaps a major element in creating alternating phases of attraction and repulsion, which express a kind of trial-and-error process that ultimately creates intention and organized behavior. All cell and tissue "behavior" is based upon constantly changing trials of exchange and interaction that manifest themselves in a well-established periodicity.

The organized movement of extracellular matrix (the fundamental substance) is dependent upon a subtle combination of a multiplicity of functional rhythms, which are displayed by:

- the endothelium of the capillaries
- circulatory changes in warmth convection
- oscillation of molecules in the fundamental substance
- transmembranous exchanges of electrolytes
- intra- and extracellular enzymatic oscillations[3]

Electrical rhythms are probably supported by spontaneous Ca^{2+}-oscillations at the cellular level, as described by Lakatta [8] in his research on the origin of heart contractility.

The osteopath should remember that a great part of the origin of rhythm is intrinsically related to biochemistry and biophysics, and that the rhythm that is sensed is not attributable to one single source, but rather to a summation of different biological origins. In other words, the fluid and its intimate relationship to the fascia rather are the vectors of rhythms, instead of the intrinsic source of rhythm. Thus, for the osteopath, the fluid and fascia should be considered as a tool rather than a source.

In accepting this hypothesis, we also accept that fluid rhythm and fasciae could increase the diagnostic field for the therapist, because they could indicate deeper concentrated layers of disturbed

---

[3] Myocytes display a "myogenic" rhythm dependent upon rhythmical ATP synthesis in the walls of the small capillaries, which express balanced phases of contraction and relaxation.

7

exchange. This means that the physical interpretation of rhythms (eg, cycles, amplitude, and strength of pulsation) contains an indication of biological integrity or disturbance.

This generation of rhythm occurs in the same way during embryological development; the fluids "drive" the cells to their final destination and structure. This drive is guaranteed by production of hyaluronic acid, which increases extracellular fluid concentration, and it is facilitated by the interaction between certain morphogens and growth factors and by the induced tissue or cell clusters. Once structure and form become firm and offer resistance, the fluids start to participate in the vectoring of a rhythm that is imposed by the restriction field. It is logical to assume that when resistance increases, fluids have to adapt and express an alteration in rhythm (ie, wavelength, frequency, power propagation of a wave pattern).

7.3 Physiological properties integrated in the vital field of the fascia

Different qualities of exchange between tissue and its inner and outer environment are expressed as integrated modalities of physiology.

7.3.1 Fluidic rhythm

The spontaneous changing states of viscosity of the tissue itself are generated by polarization and depolarization of cells in the ECM. Changes in membranous tension create altering states of concentration of the ECM (ie, more solutes are found in the ECM) and dilution of the ECM (ie, fewer solutes are found). These two phases are known as the sol phase and the gel phase. They determine the state of strength of a tissue, which could be qualified as the "tonicity" of the tissue.

The main mechanism is a transmembranous exchange of electrolytes, creating a kind of "solvent drag" that either concentrates or dilutes different kinds of molecules outside or inside the cell environment.

Fluid exchange and electrical fields in tissue seem mutually interdependent. Other fluid exchanges could perhaps support, or be partially dependent upon, this basic hydroelectrical state of the tissue.

Exchanges between the arterial-venous vascular bed and the lymphatic circulation codetermine part of the rhythmic expression of the fascial environment. It is possible that the rhythm expressed by the lymphatic bed is dependent upon an intrinsic rhythm of the vascular wall of the vein.[4] [9] In addition, fluid exchanges between the lymphatic bed and the ECM, or between the CSF and the cortical veins, have to be considered as potential generators of rhythm in the body.

7.3.2 The fascia as a pulsating field

The fascia, as an outer and inner envelop of the body, can be considered as a huge, widespread field that receives at each place of its anatomical organization the impact of the heart by means of its arterial pulsation. The quality of this fluidic shock is an appreciable tool in evaluating local resistance of the tissue, and by this means also a possible transmitter of organized pathology.

Traditional Chinese medicine has long used the quality of the peripheral heartbeat for evaluating organic disease or health. Classic Western medicine mentions the value of an exaggerated heart pulse, either visible or palpable, as a useful tool in diagnosing some diseased states. Visible heartbeat in the epigastric region of the abdomen can be considered as an indicator of advanced enteroptosis of the viscera. Palpable and deviated heartbeat in the epigastric region can be considered as an indicator of possible aortic or renal aneurysm.

The well-trained osteopath should be able to recognize any alteration in pulse strength as a possible indicator of a changed local trophic state of tissue

---

4 The rhythm found in the venous wall displays a pattern of approximately 12 pulsations/minute. Lymphatic propulsion expresses this same pattern. Thus, one could hypothesize that the basic rhythm of the body may be transmitted by the rhythm contained in the omphalomesenteric veins that link the vital field of the mother to that of the embryo.

(eg, fibrotic tissue) or as an expression field of more centralized and organic disease.

7.3.3 The fascia as a frequency-integrating field

The fascia is obedient to the laws of atomic dynamics and displacement. Particles, expressing a certain velocity and force while hitting a surface, add a certain quantum of energy to the substrate of the surface. This energy will be transformed into a transmission or flux characteristic for the cell population composing the substrate.

• A light ray will enter the eye and transfer its frequency to the retina, which, being hit by particular photons, transforms this mechanical energy into electrical impulses. The impulses convey activating or inhibiting messages to the optic nerve. This messaging is transformed in different cortical domains into specific visual images that are interpreted by the striata, peristriata, and parastriata areas of the occipital cortex.

• A sound wave hits the tympanic diaphragm and is translated and conveyed by osseous tissue and fluid to the acoustic nerve, which retranslates the message by means of electrical waves to the acoustic (temporal) area. There, the individual can interpret words and meanings of the message by combining the received information with other information stored in the convergence zones of the cortex.

• Gaseous solutions of odors are accelerated by air streams passing over the superior conchae of the nose, and they make contact with a nasal field where the gas molecules are integrated in the mucosal covering of this sensory area. There, they are transformed into electrical impulses and transmitted by the mitral cells into the olfactory bulb. The impulses are conveyed to the lateral, intermediate, and medial olfactory areas that are specific for olfactory integration and interpretation (uncus, entorhinal area, limen insula, amygdaloid body, anterior perforated area, septal area). [10, 11]

These transmissions of energy are probably the most specific and best known. Nevertheless, other physical interactions between energy and matter exist and suggest a polyvalence of certain tissues in transmitting sources of physical energy. Not all transitions of energy in the brain are bound to electrochemical ways of transmission. For example, some are also dependent upon electrotonical transmission.

Experiments conducted with sound transmission on the fascia superficialis of the body demonstrate the capability of this tissue for nonspecific sound transmission, which can be partly interpreted by the auditory apparatus of the body. This phenomenon has been described as "neurophonia".

It seems reasonable to accept that the skin and this fascia superficialis can sense the intensity of air streams. We believe that the skin covering the face and scalp is very sensitive to such air displacements because its sensitive afference is intimately integrated in the cranial nerve circuit, between the fifth and seventh cranial nerves. These nerves simultaneously govern motor impulses and integrate other neurosensorial and behavioral impulses in their own trajectories.

7.3.4 A most subtle mechanical tension field governing tissue and fluidic tonuses

Oxygen molecules combined with gaseous hydrogen are capable of creating a surface tension of liquid origin, which is used by sugar biopolymers in their function as constructors or destroyers. The body fluid may be considered as the most basic organizer of body tension.

Based on this point of view, it is not so astonishing that one finds a correlation between the degree of hydration of the body and the acute and paroxystic events that inhibit normal physiology. Dehydration from severe diarrhea can organize an acute lumbago; local swelling can inhibit normal mobility of a particular joint. One could suppose that most of these paroxysms are programmed by deep-lying unbalanced exchanges at the hydroelectrolytic level.

7.3.5 The fascia as a light captor

One of the most intriguing questions one can ask concerns how life, as a vital impulse, is transmitted.

Even if we understand much about the biochemical and biophysical transmitters of cellular and molecular energy, the question remains: should we conceive of the origin of energy inside or outside the body?

By studying the evolutionary phases of cell maturation and tissue development, one can note that neural crest cells and their migrations govern a great deal of the functional exchange of the embryonic body besides genetic patterning. This happens in a brief time scale covering the first four to eight weeks of development. These cells transform themselves into melanin-bearing cells that migrate to the superficial tissue layers of the body (fascia superficialis), as if they are conditioned to organize and captivate light impulses. These same events occur in the migration of the optic nerve fibers, where melanin-bearing cells may be necessary to act as guides. [12]

It could be hypothesized that all fasciae, especially the superficial fasciae, function in various gradations as light captors that activate and intensify vital processes in the body. We could propose that fasciae transmit exogenous energy sources into integrative physiological levels, where they translate and communicate these energy balances by complex interdigitated myofascial and organofascial continuity. Furthermore, these same pathways transmit endogenous energy balances.

Schematizing the physical events that influence the fasciae could lead to the following proposals:

- Light displays a frequency that carries a "certain load," which, when hitting a specialized tissue appropriately, prefers a liquid environment (even mucus) for integration and intensification of this energy transmission.
- Another part of energy transmission happens by bony or diaphragmlike structures, such as the acoustic tympanum.
- The transmission of energy will result in reorganization of the electrical field from the exited tissue, which will be interpreted by specialized and centralized tissue as a specific message.
- The changes in frequency and in electrical field density of the tissue are capable of reorganizing and reorienting tissue structure and exchange. This can be perceived by appropriate palpation.
- The tissue is the force plate into which subtle energies (eg, light frequencies, sound waves, gaseous solutions) are transformed into much more

dense properties, such as strength, tonus, orientation, fixation, and molecular exchanges. In this process, the addition of energy (thixotropic effect) is capable of altering tissue and cellular integrative and transformative capacities.
- The palpating hand can perceive different qualities of tissue information.

D. Bois [4] describes different mechanical and rhythmical qualities for palpatory information:

- Ether movement can be perceived as pulsating.
- Liquid displacement is sensed as fluctuation or as pulsation.
- Membranes are expressing impulses.
- Bone expresses rhythmical changes when one palpates joint play.

We hope it is now clear that the fascia, including the whole connective tissue, can transmit a much broader array of diagnostic subtleties than the purely mechanical and physical aspects of diagnosis.

7.4 Brief embryological considerations

A.T. Still proposed that the womb is almost a complete being in and of itself. He described it as the center, the origin, and the mother of all fasciae. He also underlined the fact that by means of the fascia, the material man is born. [1] In fact, the entire process of structuring and orientating tissue and its specific functions seems to be dependent upon two major cellular dynamics: ecto-mesenchymal interactions and epithelio-mesenchymal interactions, or transitions (the same as the EMT's previously mentioned).

EMT's start very early in embryonic life, during the late blastula/early gastrula stage. These EMT's first appear as epiblast cell transformations that display as bottle cells. These cells ingress at the primitive streak and the node, functioning as a starting signal for a series of tissue transformations and organogenesis (➤ Fig 7.3). In addition, the neural crest cells (NCC's) can be considered as a type of EMT at the borders of the closing neural groove. They function as precursors for well-defined cell specifications, sometimes at a considerable distance from their origin (discussed later in the text).

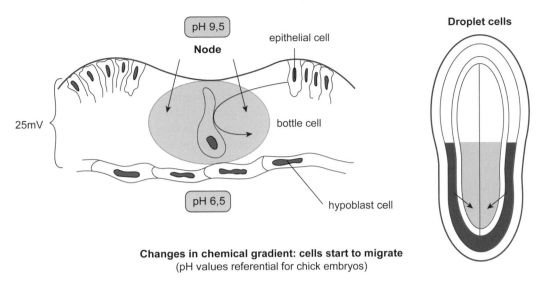

Changes in chemical gradient: cells start to migrate
(pH values referential for chick embryos)

Fig. 7.3 Differences in pH gradients between the amniotic side and the coelomic side of the embryo are considered to be important for creating a microvoltage gradient, which could support oriented migration of bottle cells and facilitation of epithelio-mesenchymal transitions.

The mesenchymal cell profiles itself as one of the most dynamic and intelligent cellular transitions throughout embryological and fetal development. It continues to be so during postnatal life, though the cell at that point has become more specific and acts as a fibroblast, a lymphocytic, or a mesothelial cell.

In the earliest stages of embryology, the mesenchymal cell functions as an articulating cell between the early epiblast and hypoblast layers. In fact, one can consider the mesenchymal cell as a transformed epiblastic cell that can display two faculties in later processing. These faculties are as the main constructor of the mesoderm layer or as a wanderer crossing the whole body as a neural crest cell.

This cell obeys and contributes to the basic laws of embryological development:

- Structure and function are basically supported by electrophysiological exchange.
- Primary structure and function are interdependent and represent nourishing currents that interact via transmembranous transport of metabolites.
- Thermal gradients are dependent on molecular frictions and collisions, mechanical interference of tissues of different origins, and differences in regional vascularization.

- Spaces are formed by differences in growth velocity between two fields, and they are always supported by EMT's and mesodermal differentiation. Spaces are necessary for organs to take their proper places and assume their correct functions. Spaces are also needed by mesodermal structures (fasciae and aponeuroses), which support and orient the integrity of each organ and of the whole body organization. For example, the interpleural space allows for negative or positive pleural tension, lung parenchyma expansion, and, finally, gaseous exchange)
- Degradation and disappearance of currents and cells occurs via apoptosis.

Part of the function of cells is vanishing during the subsequent periods of embryological and fetal development. In a sense, they serve in "trial-and-error" events that help to support essential phases of function.

One can suppose that during this processing, cells go through a period of gradual "learning,"[5] and that part of their function can be recapitulated during the urgent adaptation needs of a specific cell population

---

[5] For example, this learning process is well established for the lymphocytic cell population.

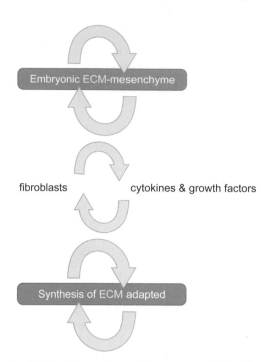

Fig. 7.4 Cytokines and growth factors secreted during fibroblast activation are important in definitive differentiation of embryonic mesenchyme in extracellular matrix (ECM) into fully functional mesenchyme serving subsequent stages of tissue maturation and differentiation.

or tissue. An example of such a need is wound healing. In another example, the cells may transform themselves into wanderer cells that form metastases in other tissues, as is the case for melanocytes.

It is possible that, because these cells bear a certain memory (➤ Fig 7.4), they remain linked to certain time-space developmental periods of embryological, fetal, perinatal, and postnatal life—periods in which the brain was also learning. The feedback mechanisms to the brain from different types of tissues are multiple. These mechanisms may proceed by means of hormonal, molecular, or peptidergic messaging, as well as by subtle changes in the frequencies arriving at receptive sites of the brain for image building.[6] [13]

An appropriate stimulus, such as shock or trauma, could activate a certain state of "cell panic," in which the self/nonself recognition of the body is disturbed. This state could induce immune and auto-immune overreactions, as described by C.W. Cotman and colleagues. [14] These overreactions might be preceded by a more silent phase, during which the body is collecting the whole array of conscious and subconscious information connected to a specific tissue or space-time.

The brain probably fabricates a complex model of integration of these multiple bits of information and decides whether it has to initiate an altered program. On a biochemical level, this program is governed by complex neurologic-endocrine-immune responses, which can establish behavioral disorders and complex immune disorders.

One could hypothesize that every inflammatory or immunological reactivity is based on adapted and integrated forms of learning. This is probably the key reason that traumatic events (both physical and psychological) can liberate an uncontrolled part of the patients' subconscience.

Subtle changes in stress adaptation or behaviors can be precious indicators of underlying altered adaptation patterns. The connective tissue is one of the omnipresent collectors of trauma-induced changes in physiology. The wide range of its cell diversity and specialization makes it an ideal matrix for pathological integration and altered retrocontrol expression. At each of their particular levels, astrocytes, macrophages, and lymphocytes display remarkable features of integrating neurochemical and endocrine messaging between the brain and the immune system.

When we examine the various embryological episodes, we could propose that the insertion of the fertilized ovum into the endometrium is a test of articulation between two foreign tissues. During its wandering through the fallopian tube and later in the womb, the fertilized ovum is guided by only one purpose: the need to find a reliable and constant source of oxygen and sugar supply.

Most life events are organized by the basic needs of searching for food and oxygen. It is no wonder that circulation and sugar saturation of the blood play important roles in guiding the fertilized ovum, or blastocyst, to insert itself into the mucosal surface

___

[6] K. Pribam defines the dendrodendritic fields in the cerebral cortex as specific receptive fields that function in a top-down, corticofugal manner and organize the images used by the brain. Pribam KH. *Brain and Perception*. New York, NY: Psychology Press, 2011: 4-11.

of the uterus. For the blastocyst, there is only one exact place to insert itself. This particular area will become the first on/off-signaling place for further vital events and exchanges.

Warmth, glucose and oxygen concentration direct the insertion of the blastocyst, guided by the quantity and quality of estrogen concentration in circulation at the womb. The therapist who succeeds in installing sufficient blood supply and, consequently, enough glucose concentration in a tissue inhibited by a traumatic incident probably supports the on-switching signal of that tissue. Wasn't this the thesis of A.T. Still when he stated, *"The law of artery is supreme"*?

In this manner, it is possible for the osteopath to treat the embryo or fetus across the belly of the pregnant woman. Slight manual sustained compression upon the area that covers the womb suffices to increase reactive blood supply in the depth of the womb and to increase exchanges between mother and child. Nature—in this case, physiology—will translate the mechanical impulse of compression or fascial technique into an adapted biochemical reactive pattern.

The osteopath who understands the laws of EMT's and mesenchymal adaptation can rely upon one of the deepest and earliest patterns of tissue organization. These patterns can be used by the body as reactive patterns to reorganize and adapt tissue to inflammatory, infectious, and traumatic events. This tissue can also be used as a motile, interactive connection between different functions and organ areas. When the osteopath applies the appropriate physical laws of tissue physiology—such as through adjustment of manual synchronization—the mesenchyme will be readjusted correctly.

This is called the balanced state of tissue adaptation or—as described by W.G. Sutherland—balanced membranous or ligamentous tension. Understanding and achieving this balance implies knowledge of the eliciting circumstance that made the tissue adapt to a nonphysiological pattern (or trauma), leading to the expression of a progressive deterioration of its structure and function. Achieving this balance also implies additional knowledge—of the eliciting circumstance's relationship to tissue patterning and reaction, of the imaging of the circumstance by the brain, and of the integration of past and present space/time schedules in the development of the morbid state of the body.

7.5 Function of the fascia related to its connection with the metabolic fields during embryogenesis

The fascia, especially in its histological constitution, can present two different states of organization. At one time, it can function as a dilated, expanded metabolic field or mesenchymal tissue, making exchanges with its environment through mechanical, hydroelectrical, and chemical parameters. At another time, it can function as a dense, concentrated tissue, such as an organ, fulfilling a specific metabolic function involving strength and elasticity.

The following example may clarify this concept. The mesothelial layer of the peritoneum can play an important role as an ultrafiltrator of fluids in its dilated state—that is, as a simple fascial, mesothelial sheet. However, it also takes part in the constitution of a more specialised organ for ultrafiltration of fluids by constructing the envelopes of perirenal spaces. The fascia's role in fluid balance of the body:

- It governs the metabolic environment of the body by serving as an exchange surface for oncotic and osmotic equilibration of body fluids.
- Its role in the Donnan effect and other physical phenomena depends on the hydroelectrical forces that are sustained by ionic exchange.
- It generates a subtle equilibrium in the extracellular and intracellular fluid balance.
- It functions as a condensed organ for control of the fluid balance of the body, as specified by the kidneys. The nephron is a concentrated condition of the preceding mesothelial function of the peritoneum during embryogenesis.
- It possesses its own control mechanism for fluid exchange, controlled by a hormonal feedback system that relates important organs of the body participating in the fluid equilibrium.

The angiotensin-renin-aldosterone coupling sustains fluid homeostasis in the body and is governed by the kidneys. At least three organs interfere to assure competent feedback for the adjustment of the renin liberation—the heart, liver, and kidneys. Dependent upon changes in pH values (chemoreceptors) and volemic pressure values (baroreceptors), these organs activate a complex nervous efferent system that

7

modifies and/or activates glomerular filtration rate and renal blood flow.

The heart (atrial natriuretic peptide),[7] the liver (angiotensin), and the kidneys (renin) elaborate a complex feedback system that is coupled to the CNS to exert control over the sympathetic nerve activity of the kidneys. [15, 16] The efferent renal sympathetic nerve activity (ERSNA) and afferent renal sympathetic nerve activity (ARSNA) govern the subtle equilibrium between chemosensitive and baroreceptive impulses.

This relationship is not only a matter of hormonal-endocrine information exchange. The fascial environment, which constitutes and envelops these three organs, actively participates in elaborating a complex biochemical and biomechanical exchange field. In addition, the brain (brain natriuretic peptide)[8], the lungs, and the intestines contribute to a lesser extent to this kind of homeostasis.

7.5.1 Contribution to hydrostatic pressure values

The heart assures and integrates the laws of the pressure/volume relationship. The Bayliss-Starling law determines part of the cardiac output, but a great deal of cardiac power is governed by the laws of elasticity of its organizing tissues. The pericard and myocard play important roles in the elastic recoil of the heart. Their integrity assures a fluctuating equilibrium between the end-systolic muscular recoil and the end-diastolic volume.

Hydrostatic pressure equilibrium is important in regulating arterial-venous capillary exchange values. This equilibrium also plays the role of a mechanical component, tensing the tiny fascial envelopes in such a way that they become a mechanical support for other physiological faculties. For example, the hydrostatic pressure in the salivary glands helps to support the myofascial tension of the lingual musculature by tensing the suprahyoidal fasciae and muscles. [17]

The **heart** represents the condensed organ for control of the hydrostatic pressure balance of the body. The liver and, to a lesser degree, the kidneys contribute to elaborate a functional hydrostatic pressure, which enables the whole body to resist gravitational forces. The same can be asserted for any anatomical and physiological level of exchange. The lungs, as well as the intestines and the brain, depend upon equilibrated pressure values to display sufficient gaseous or molecular exchange essential for their physiology.

Intercalated between the dense organs and the vascular domain are all the tissues that interfere with, or are intimately dependent upon, hydrostatic pressure changes. The vascular tissue, as well as all kinds of interstitial tissue, must be examined for their properties of liberty of exchange. To understand the importance of the mesentery's integrity for fluid homeostasis in the body, it suffices to mention that the mesentery on its own can be considered as one of the most important vascular (venous) "spare tanks" of the body. Its importance lies in vascular-lymphatic exchange.

The lymph could be described as an end product of the exchange between the vascular and the extracellular field. It could further be considered as a concentration of blood plasma and extracellular fluid. In a certain way, it is a fluidic articulation that refers to the homeostatic level of the body in its exchange with its environment (metabolic, mechanical, and neuroendocrine movements). The physical laws that govern these fluid motions and support their subtle exchanges are dependent upon the concentrations of different macro- and micromolecules. These molecules organize the oncotic pressure and transmembraneous exchange (Donnan effect) of fluids.

The organ that constitutes the "masterpiece" in generating lymphatic pressure is the **liver.** This large gland is able to increase its daily lymph production from about 1.5 L to 10-15 L and to destabilize normal volume values of the body.

Ascites is the usual "adaptive" pathological pattern found during dramatic increases of portal pressure. Subtle edematous changes may be found at distances from the site of portal hypertension (eg, inguinal region), indicating a more profound suffering of the metabolic area. The liver, spleen, and heart constitute the functional triad that governs the

---

consequence of portal hypertension. The more "loose," flaccid, and mobile organ is represented by the peritoneum, which plays the role of generator and integrator of ascites.

7.5.2 Role in immune-lymphatic equilibrium

Some remarkable cellular immunological activities are dependent upon the integrity of reactive and adaptive tissues, such as the vascular walls and the reticular endothelial tissue. These tissues, together with most of the loose connective tissue, represent and support the embryological cellular migrations that organize much of the space/time relationship of the body and its structure. According to this concept, the tissue not only participates in the formation of an immune memory, but it is also the condensed site of these immunological activities. The mesenchyme, again, seems to be the excellent integrator of these "memories." [18]

It suffices to study the development of the immunological system during embryogenesis to understand that the precursor lymphocytes display great migratory facility in reaching the condensed area of the thymus anlage to germinate. The **thymus** is the best expression of a focalised "informative" area that integrates different cellular migrations to realise its properties as a germination center.

Neural crest information, as well as vascular sprouting, are necessary to facilitate the thymus's function as an immunological "force plate." [19] The functional triad at this specific immunological level is represented by the germination layers in the thymus, bone marrow, and spleen (Schweigger-Seidel sheath).

All mesenchyme-derived envelopes of the thymus, bone marrow, spleen, and liver relate this topographically distributed immune memory to the vascular-humoral propagated immune response.

7.5.3 Relation to the biomechanical level

It is clear that myofascial tensions disturb the normal postural adaptive capacity of the body. The **parietal muscle,** in its aerobic and anaerobic energy expansion, is related to the hemodynamic force of the *heart*. It is similarly related to the metabolic force of the *liver*, to metabolise muscle energy. The hydroelectrical tension displayed by the liver is largely dependent upon an intact *kidney* function. One could propose that if any of these three organs becomes exhausted, it would be normal to loose muscle energy and, consequently, muscle force.

The metabolic, hydrostatic, and hydroelectric values are sensed and adapted in a widespread fascial and myofascial field that surrounds and relates different muscle units. Dysfunction of a fascia—by fibrosis, inflammation, or congestion—disturbs normal energy expenditure and could serve as a disabling memory unit for normal muscular and postural expression. Fatigue and muscle weakness should be treated by deparalyzing the fascia and by strengthening the organs.

7.5.4 Relation to the brain

Two sentences from A.T. Still reveal the importance of the fascia for the integrity of brain function: *"The fascia is the branch office of the brain. Why not treat these branch offices with the same respect as the brain?"*

The fascial tissue functions as an articulation between the central and peripheral nervous systems. Any intelligent osteopath should know that the slightest fixation of the central and peripheral fascial pathways could inhibit normal transmission of neuronal signalling. Most of these pathways have been organized during embryogenesis, and they constitute an important referential pattern for adaptive and integrative behavior.

We may suggest that any change in the episodic homeostatic adaptation of the body—whether it succeeds or fails—is supported by a particular fascial facilitation or inhibition.

REFERENCES
[1] Still AT. The Philosophy and Mechanical Principles of Osteopathy. Reprint. Kirksville, MO: Osteopathic Enterprise, 1986:60–61.
[2] Barral JP, Mercier P. Manipulations viscérales. Vol 1. Paris, France: Elsevier Masson, 1983.

[3] Roques M, Gabarel B. Les fasciae en medicine osteo-pathique. Vol 1. Paris, France: Maloine, 1985:31–101.

[4] Bois D. Concepts fondamentaux de fasciathérapie et de pulsologie profonde. Paris, France: Maloine, 1984:17–26.

[5] Wheather R, Burkitt HG. Histologie fonctionelle. Paris, France: Medsi/McGraw Hill, 1987.

[6] Pischinger A. Das System de Grundregulation. 7th ed. Heidelberg, Germany: Haug Verlag, 1985.

[7] Upledger J. Craniosacral Therapy II: Beyond the Dura. Seattle, WA: Eastland Press, 1987.

[8] Lakatta EG. Functional implications of spontaneous sarcoplacmic reticulum Ca2+ release in the heart. Cardiovasc Res. 1992;26(3):193–214.

[9] Farasyn A. Nouvelle hypothèse sur la cause du mouvement crânien. Journées belges de médicine ostéopathique. Paper presented at: Symposium, Faculté de sciences, Université de Namur; January 18, 1986; Namur, Belgium.

[10] Clos J, Muller Y. Neurobiologie cellulaire. Vol 2. Paris, France: Nathan, 1997.

[11] Wilson-Pauwels L, et al. Cranial Nerves. Hamilton, ON: BC Decker, 1988.

[12] Witkop CJ, et al. Optic and otic neurological abnormalities in oculocutaneous and ocular albinism. Birth Defects. 1982;18(6):299–318.

[13] Pribram KH. Brain and Perception: Holonomy and Structure in Figural Processing. New York, NY: Routledge, 2011:4–11.

[14] Cotman CW, et al. The Neuro-Immune-Endocrine Connection. New York, NY: Raven Press, 1987:71–92.

[15] DiBona GF, Kopp UC. Neural control of renal function. Physiol Rev. 1997;77(1):75–197.

[16] O'Hagan KP, et al. Cardiac receptors modulate the renal sympathetic response to dynamic exercise in rabbits. J Appl Physiol. 1994;76(2):507–515.

[17] Homberger DG, Meyers RA. Morphology of the lingual apparatus of the domestic chicken, Gallus gallus, with special attention to the structure of the fasciae. Am J Anat. 1989;186(3):217–257.

[18] Dubreuil G. Embryologie humaine. Paris, France: Vigot, 1947:202.

[19] Bockman DE, Kirby ML. Dependence of thymus development on derivatives of the neural crest. Science. 1984;223(4635):498–500.

7

CHAPTER

8 Body memory and the original lesion

8.1 Philosophical considerations

Is the whole body constantly functioning through tests of adaptations, or does it simultaneously create definitive modifications in its physical environment? Is homeostasis a labile or a stable expression of physiological equilibrium? In other words, does the body need transient stages of allostasis for finding an adapted equilibrium upon constantly changing circumstances?

We could consider the allostatic episodes as adaptive "swipes" that upregulate the integrative capability of the body, if the episodes are not too long-lasting or aggressive. They could lead to a more appropriate state of adaptation of the body upon the changing character of the inner and outer environment. Apparently, the human body, as any other structure, is the product of the constant adaptation to external influences and the intrinsic physiological capabilities to do so.

The entire morphogenesis can be regarded as a succession of adaptations of embryonic tissues to the stress-shifts caused by external influences. [1] We function as "fractals" of adaptive energy that modify, in an invisible way, our physical field of interaction and the layout of our impulses. According to this view, we are rather passive fields, activated by appropriate stimuli that correspond largely to a programmed probability. We are programmed to get old, grey, bald, and sick, and to die—and perhaps also to get wealthy, famous, and wise.

A rhetorical question emerges: What is the advantage of being rich and famous when you are dead? First, consider that the programming and readaptation to newer incoming information in the immune field is analogous to that in the cognitive field. Then compare the use of such constant adaptations for one who is determined to get old, grey, and rich versus one who becomes merely old, grey, and poor. Do such adaptations ultimately achieve a personal goal, or are they better thought of as trangenerational adaptive trials?

The living body tests adaptations based upon intrinsic integrative capabilities. It integrates various kinds of stimuli—but it also emits purposes, and it verifies part of its emission in a conscious way. [2] We can calculate and estimate the efficiency of purposes, and we call it probability and statistics.

A great part of what the human brain emits is referential, and we call it science. We calculate the probabilities of space and time necessary to cross and to transgress them. We create new concepts about time and space, and we reach the limits of quantum theory. We find time space units without constant form, and we touch the border of chaos. In the best possible case, we might discover a rhythm and identify some patterns.

Many paradigmatic questions arise.

Could we call chaos the "starting point," or entropy the "motion point" or a "constant hyperbole of transition between visible and invisible energy transition forms"? Are chaos and the patterns that evolve from it the formless parts of consciousness?[1] Could it be that the subconscious is more chaotic and also freer than the conscious? Am I sane because I am consciously interacting with reality, or is it my subconscious that tries to break free from the conscious and to achieve fixed purposes and convictions through awareness?

Most likely, the subconscious tries to free itself from firmly fixed space-time units by creating impulses, which confront us with our limitations.

Don't we all try to get free, to live free, and to eliminate obstacles that limit our free movement?

---

[1] It is considered as almost evident that chaos spontaneously leads to structuration and patterning.

Again, a rhetorical question arises: Is the study of a form a science or an ideology? A more immediately question is: Is an object, whether scientific or ideological, a representation of freedom or an expression of unrecognized restriction of exchange?

The question of whether form, in any gradation of subtlety, is an independent feature or a self-limiting memory can be quickly resolved by the following considerations.

Any form seems to be built upon a specific time-space unit and expresses the "freedom" of its potential in range-specific physical and behavioral patterns. For the human being, the physical pattern could be as "free" as his or her own body consciousness is sophisticated. The freedom of the behavioral pattern may be represented by the limitations we experience in the emotional, affective, and intellectual fields. Intelligence includes, in this context, a certain paradigm: the more the intellectual knowledge progresses, the more the restriction becomes unbearable, inviting behavioral events that lead to freedom.

Allow me to refer to an old Chinese proverb: *"The one who detains a prisoner gets captured himself."* In other words, the one who clings to a conviction becomes dependent upon it.

Life seems to be the echo of the subconscious reflected in the desire for comprehension by human intelligence:

- Intelligence strives for control.
- The subconscious strives for freedom.
- Life, through progressive adaptations, struggles for stillness as the ultimate condition that favors healing or reintegration of health in the body.

In the osteopathic concept, some authors go beyond life to define the origin of memory—and that of health. Health *"underpins the order of all structure and function within the human system."* [3] Health is defined as the *"blueprint energy,"* as an *"original matrix,"* or—in the words of Sutherland when he taught how to direct the Tide [4] (the movement of fluids concentrated around the body's midline)—as "intelligence with a capital I." Memory seems to lie beyond the conventional memory that neurologists localize in the brain; it lies even beyond cellular memory.[2] Memory is like an informative power that

emerges from a common frequency field or light field that unlocks the enclosed potential of the genome, activating the essence of life within a range of probabilities enclosed in the genetic code.

To be more descriptive, memory is like a quantum code plucking the strings of DNA [5] and freeing the intrinsic capability of a probable interaction with transient energy fields. That interaction will determine part of the space/time scale of the transforming consciousness, which is expressed in a constantly changing form. [6]

"The geometric configuration of the human body and the metabolic processes are present before the central nervous system develops... The innate wisdom in the body is not contained within any cellular structure." [3]

The ultimate memory is wisdom and health, not destabilized in their integrative capacity by any disturbing information. But it was A.T. Still who proclaimed that it is easier to find disease than to find health. Symbolically, the body expresses its wisdom through the "midline function." The midline around which the human body develops includes the first functions to appear in our physical organization. *These functions include the molecular, cellular, tissue, and organ physiologies.* [3]

The midline serves as the memory of ultimate balancing. It is an ever-memorized momentum to which each specific cell or function has a natural tendency to strive. All molecules of the body "know" about their polarity in relation to the midline. That is why Sutherland gave so much attention to directing the Tide: *"Don't exert any power upon the Tide, trust upon it."*

The Tide seems to be the expression of the subtle power of health. Sutherland called it "the fluid in the fluids." It is the potency of the breath of life—the vital essence—that drives the fluids, that makes them radiate outward from this midline. According to this concept, the midline is not a physical thing, but a function. Around this central function, the cellular and tissue world organizes.

The Tide generates electrical force and, therefore, determines both brain function and function of the nerves. [4] It is *"liquid light."*

In making a provisional summary, one could propose the following:

---

[2] Genes are not proactive. They are responsive. [3]

- Life, in its ultimate manifestation, is an expression of health.
- The ultimate memory is health, rather than any cerebral or cellular integration.
- Health manifests as a Tidal movement, expressing the force and depth of oceanic sound and movement—that is, a dull watery sound suggestive of great depth and unknown power.

The breath of life is vitalized and organized in this Tidal movement.

- The Tide manifests and organizes life around a midline function.
- Every cellular and organic physiology seems orientated around this midline function.
- The deepest tendency of the cell, tissue, and body is to preserve health by balancing, as closely as possible, around this midline function.
- Every physiology expresses a midline function, a point of "balanced tension."
- Memory in the human system is a balance between an initial, nondisturbed Tide and fixed points of adapted or disturbed function.
- The Tide is a memory on its own, and a diseased state is a consciousness of a disturbed Tidal movement.
- The therapeutic momentum possesses two important sequences:
  - first, the elimination of symptom and disease
  - second, the reintegration of health by directing the Tide.

The need for restoring health may be induced by the signs of illness, but health cannot be restored by eliminating illness only. A new reinforcement of the feeling of the midline function is needed before the body can remember itself and install new patterns of interference.

8.2 Stocked energy and blocked information

Embryological evolution shows how the brain, during its development, uses metabolic compounds to construct a one-way metabolic field before elaborating specific neural pathways that express neurological function. During the first episode of organogenesis, the blood becomes the main path by which metabolites are conveyed to the brain. The heart becomes the force plate (or turning point) for the metabolic trains to and from the brain. The information from the liver passes through the heart and gets stocked and structured in the brain.

The first way of stocking, displayed by brain tissue during organogenesis, is a modulating of metabolic information into formative processes that structure and organize the anatomy and topography of the brain areas. After the brain becomes an elaborated neurological center, it starts to emit electrical impulses guided in semiliquid tubes (ie, the perineurium of the nerves). The progression of liquid in the perineural tubes is prolonged initially into the envelopes wrapped around the collagen tubes of its own fasciae (the dural membranes) and ultimately into the peripheral fasciae throughout the body. Transmission of a signal seems to be more than a neurological impulse; it is also organic and biochemical.

One can also note that the information on both sides of the integrative fields—the brain and periphery—passes over specific biochemical and fluidic pathways. It is first integrated in a general metabolic field before becoming a specific neurological message. In other words, metabolic information is first integrated in the brain substrate. Afterwards, part of this information is reconstituted to the periphery under specific fluidic and electrical patterns.

Both parts, the center and the periphery, can stimulate and inhibit each other in two ways:
- by specific neurological programming
- by subjacent "background information" passing into the vast area of cellular, tissue, and fluidic exchange.

The background information forms the basic "tune" upon which normal neurological development proceeds. In some cases, the information is blocked in the brain, and the energy remains concentrated in the visceral domain. In other cases, the information is stocked in the periphery, and the energy transmission is inhibited in the brain. Only inhibitory and facilitating fascial testing between the two areas permits us to elucidate origin and symptom.

As a preliminary conclusion, we could propose that a brain dysfunction can find its origin in the visceral parts of the body, and that a visceral dysfunction can be induced by brain "shortcuts." One has to

8

understand that the brain is *a part of the body,* and that the body is *an integrated image* in the brain that can be used to organize whole body function, including brain function.

Yet, too often, the brain is treated and considered as the highest level of autonomy. One has to remember that a sick body creates, in most cases, a disabled brain. The holonomic viewpoint of osteopathy makes it impossible for the therapist to separate brain function from body function.

8.3 Memorization inside and outside matter

- Science accepts the concept of *a neuroendocrine type of memory.*
  This memory is apparently localized in the archaic structures of the hippocampal circumvolution and the limbic system. New information, passing over neuronal pathways to the nuclei of the thalamus, is projected to the outer layers of the cortex and to the circuit of Papez. [4] These complex circuits establish an intimate relationship and equilibrium between the cortical and endocrine functions. Such areas as the hippocampus and the amygdalae form the basic substrate for the integration and expression of emotions, including fear, sadness, and happiness.
- Another part of memory seems to be stocked in *the immunological circuitry.* This system is referred to as "the circulating brain." Cellular and humoral information of this kind builds a complex interference with the brain and controls the adaptive or defensive tonus of the body. B and T cells constitute the "workbench" for this type of memory.
- *Cellular memory* is encrypted in the RNA and DNA codes and in the enzymatic circuitry related to intracellular transcription modalities.
- Chromosomes are the most complex and dominant structures that transmit codes, combining them into complicated formulae that lead to the generation of new material.
- Tissue, especially *connective tissue,* possesses two major databases for storing information:

  - cell DNA, made of the bases A, C, G, and T, which can form 64 possible combinations of storage [5]
  - glucoproteins, which can encode as many as 35,560 new signals in their sugar biopolymers.
- Cytokines seem to organize a short-lasting time-space unit of information, participating in this way in the memorization of messages.
- Mechanical deformation of the connective tissue can be established as memory if the following conditions are fulfilled: [6]
  - the presence of collagen and elastin, which are serially associated during exposure to mechanical stress
  - a nonphysiological deformation of the elastin-collagen complex, not exceeding 30% of the initial length of this mechanical unit
  - the passage of a certain amount of deformation time before the information can be stored or reacted upon.

The connective tissue, by means of its link with the neuroendocrine, immunological, and biomechanical apparatus, will be able to materialize any stress—whether physical, emotional, or psychological in origin. Nothing can happen without being encrypted into the physical codons the body possesses at the very depth of its own tissue.

The preceding description of the different modalities of memory is limited to that which can be almost completely proved and evaluated in the physiological domain. This kind of memory obeys the physical laws of motion, force, resistance, and orientation of movement; otherwise life would not be adaptive. Without this adaptive capability governed by these physical laws, vitality would be a static event without significant changes and without transmutation.

The interference between the encoded program and the fluctuating environmental information creates real life modalities and expressions. [7] In this sense, rhythm, motion, and orientation express the most basic modalities of memory.

It is evident that a stiffened, inert body area or tissue can concentrate a particular memory through inflammatory processes or fibrosis. Part of the information is stocked in situ, in the tissue, and part is located in the brain. The brain is able to memorise when the tissue transmits the integrated information, but the same is possible in the inverse way.

The brain, starting with a single neuron, functions as both a captor and a servant of its physical environment from the very beginning. That means that every change in information, form, or exchange is stored somewhere in a brain unit, and this information can be shared with the actualized state of the body at some point in the future.

Pain and stress afferences follow complex routes over thalamocortical pathways and remain interconnected by different contacts in the limbic system. [8] This interference will change the rhythm, the motion, and the orientation of the vital energy of the patient's body. Tide and potency, as expressions of the individual's original life force, **may** display either a slight or a profoundly changed expressive pattern—a kind of *strain pattern*.

The tissue-cell exchange represents the balance between the cognitive aspect of memory (conscious or subconscious) and the physical-emotional-mental event that led to the memory. Even the cognitive part of memory—that which we call memorization (ie, "I remember…")—is not really the basal part of memory. Rather, it evokes, when liberated, a basic feeling. All memory and cognitive interactions are, in fact, built upon a process that progresses from sensation to feeling to awareness and, finally, to cognition.

There are two basic feelings that we can qualify as "motor": comfort and fear. [9, 10] The body knows what it means to be comfortable, because it knows what it means to be healthy. It remembers health. That's why it continually strives for a better situation—recovery or adaptation. Fear represents the possibility of perturbation of comfort. That's why fear motivates various propulsive and impulsive movements in life, including rage, envy, uncertainty, and neurotic behaviour.

Thus, we could propose that the memorizing process becomes activated when a particular situation or moment disturbs the basic feeling of comfort. And memory becomes concrete when matter focuses upon fear.

Fear could be materialized on a quantum level by the transformation of chaos into a concrete, organised form. It could be a simple movement between love and hate, between power and force, or between intelligence and intellect. When the natural chaotic state becomes disturbed in one of its qualities, matter becomes focalised and orientated. In the brain,

this condition can represent a hyperpolarized state of certain areas. These areas start to express a certain force and rhythm and a defined predisposition for interference.

Fear represents the transmutation of the natural into the restricted. In this way, anxiety becomes the balance point between the mental and physical worlds. Fear can be represented by curiosity, by envy, or by the need to know or control. It can also induce positive movements, such as science, humanity, or love.

Fear can be conceived of as a disturbing movement that interferes with the deep power of nature, the power to transform. It is the entropy state of an organized biological system that does not know the purpose of transformation. Potency and force are expressions of the inherent and silent state of nature. Pure nature does not express or even induce fear. Rather, it is an invitation to become silent.

The teachings of W.G. Sutherland and R. Becker indicate that when one has much practice in "listening" to the rhythm of the primary force, one will become increasingly focused on the "silence" in the rhythm, the silence of the movement. This can be compared with listening to a classic concerto by Bach or Mozart in which one becomes increasingly familiar with the melody by listening to the pauses in the music. The pause creates a melody in origin; the sound is accentuated by the silence that reigns. That is what R. Becker called "stillness."

Most osteopaths focus upon motion. Only after lengthy practise do they start to listen to the silence—the stillness.

Stillness could be defined as the ultimate memory, as the origin of memory, or, perhaps best, as the memory of origin (➤ Fig. 8.1). This is the kind of memory that one cannot describe with words. You have to "listen" to it, the body has to feel it, and the hands have to sense it. You know it is residing in the body, and even the body is constantly in search of it.

The following analogy might help in understanding this concept. You are sitting in a small boat on a quiet ocean when suddenly you become aware of the presence of a huge whale beneath you, deep in the ocean. You can feel this presence in the slightly different pattern of wave movement. You can't see the whale and you can't describe it verbally, but you can feel its presence through the minimal agitation of

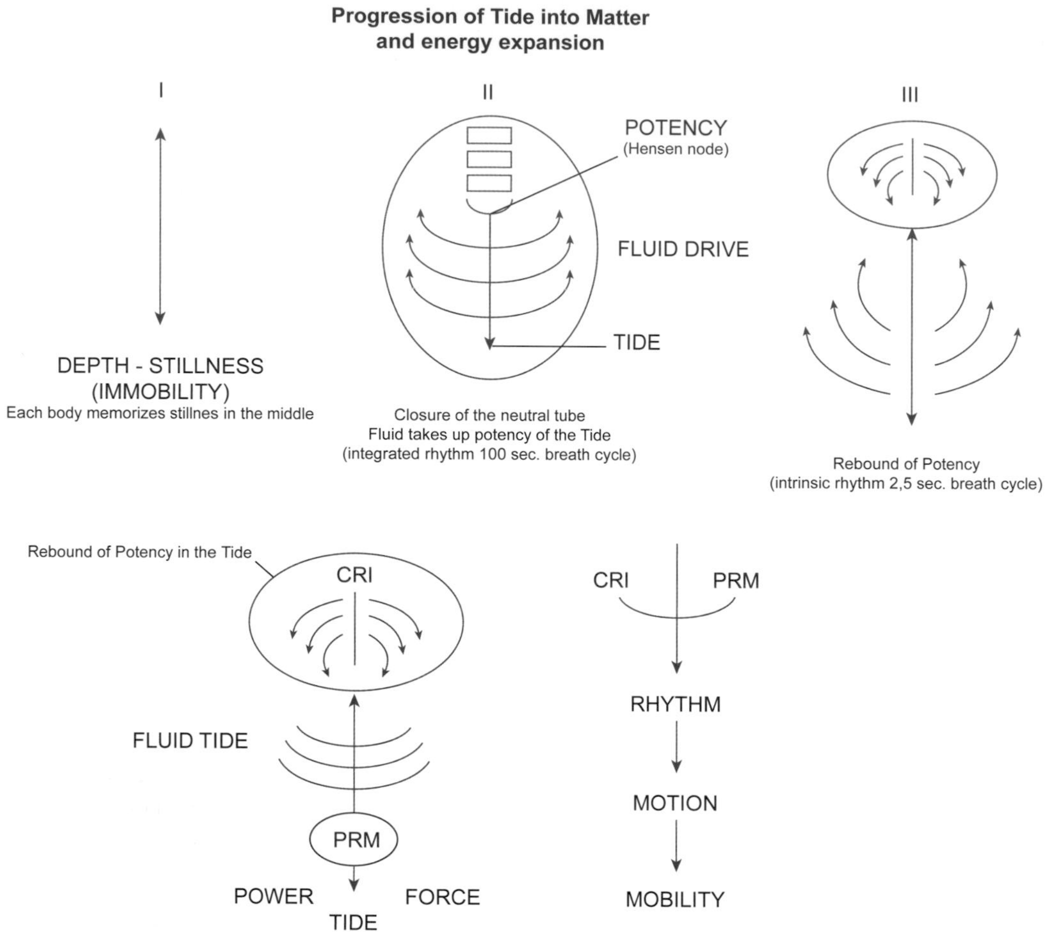

Fig. 8.1 Rhythm (cranial rhythmic impulse [CRI]) and the Tide (primary respiratory mechanism [PRM]) have both physical/quantum expression modalities and fluidal properties when propagated through the body systems. However, it is the stillness, or silence, in the rhythm that can provide the most useful information for the osteopath.

the water. You somehow have a sense that the whale is observing you without wanting to hurt you, and this sense calms you. The whale knows the depth and the width of the ocean, and he feels like the master of these waters. You presume the great depth of the ocean by the unseen presence of the whale. Although you know that the whale is there, you cannot describe his precise movements nor the precise depth where he swims. You have only this undefined feeling, and you have to accept it. Perhaps this feeling starts informing you in unknown ways.

Dr. Sutherland [11] taught us to rely upon the Tide, because it will bring us to the ultimate point of stillness. One can describe this ultimate point of

stillness as the potent place where no action is needed and where memory loses its significance.

When considering the embryo and its transformation of matter into structured form and function, it is clear that there initially exists a symmetrical structuring. The whole tissue orientation and differentiation occurs along a central line that seems to be organized outward from an "impansion pit," called Hensen's node. This node regresses in a caudal direction, and the more it regresses, the more somitomeres are built in the mesodermal central anlage (the paraxial mesoderm). These are arranged in a strict order of seven somitomeres that create the generation of one somite—a relationship of 7 to 1.

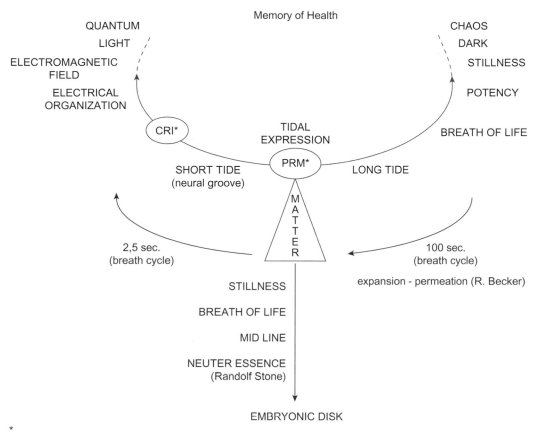

Fig. 8.2 The origin of the Tide, and its relationship to the memory of health

*
- CRI Cranial Rhytmic Impulse
- PRM Primary Respiratory Mechanism

It seems as if the somites are pushing the central line and Hensen's node backward as they themselves progress in a cranial direction. In a certain way, the cranial somites lean upon the underlying condensed mesodermal tissue. The cephalad progression and differentiation in tissue density drives a progressive compression of the caudal mesodermal anlage.

The end result is the appearance of a kind of masterpiece bone—the sacrum.

The sacral bone represents a condensed and compressed energy that encloses all possible progressions of cephalad development, from the spine to the skull. It represents primordial matter that serves to structure and direct the early tissues. It appears to be immobile in the adult, but it is not motionless. It probably represents the deepest point of stillness encoded in matter, and it informs us about the original memory and life force source, in which resides the Tide.

Another point of motionless presence lies at the top of the notochord. It appears as a referential point around which all cell "movements" take place. However, it is not actually the cells themselves that move. Rather, the cells are moved by the movement or displacement of the entire embryological body around this point of zero motion.[3]

---

[3] B. Fryman studied the integration of germinative cells along the allantois and their trajectory into the primitive mesogastrium and mesentery. He concluded that they were moved by the motion of the whole body around the top of the notochord.

Every central or lateral structure of the embryonic body is formed by subtle fluid streams, starting in the midline and flowing in a caudal-cephalad direction or in a lateral direction between the differentiated tissue sleeves. The migratory trajectories of the mesenchymal cells and neural crest cells suggest the importance of studying the dynamics of fluids and cells. Fluids and subtle exchanges between tissues and secretory cells sustain every migration. Liquefaction of the trajectories is assured by hyaluronic acid, and fibronectin traces the migratory routes.

The force of the Tide animates the fluid (➤ Fig. 8.2). In the same way that the waves of the ocean carve figures on the sand of the beach, the waves of the Tide structure the various tissue landscapes of the body and enable them to function. The fluid abuts against the restraining force of the cephalic fasciae (ectomesenchymal layer), creating motions that stop only at death.

The rhythm that is created in this way represents an ideal frequency to sustain body physiology. The fluctuation of 10 cycles/minute seems to be an ideal motion for sustaining a homeostatic exchange between tissue and fluid. Sutherland called this the cranial respiratory mechanism, or cranial respiratory impulse (CRM/CRI). It translates the rhythm, amplitude, and force of the vital breath.

Every osteopath who was motivated and astonished by the study of the cranio-sacral-sternal mechanism and the function of the core link [12] knows the rest of the story.

8.4 Tide versus trauma

Both Tide and physical shocks generate waves in the body and can influence vital energy to alter cellular frequencies. The Tide creates vital waves and rhythm. Traumatic energy creates additional shock waves, disturbing the CRM.

Dynamics similar to the vital processing of the Tide can be observed by carefully watching the motion of water after a large drop falls to the water surface in a bathtub. At first, a small crater appears at the surface of the water. Then, there is a miniscule

moment of stillness, followed by the development of an outward-spreading ripple, or wave, across the surface. The wave divides into smaller waves that display a certain rhythm. When arriving at the margin of the bathtub, the water starts quivering. Part of the quiver ends as stillness, but another part is reconstituted to the center of the water surface as a recurrent slow wave. The place where the drop entered the water surface is not the center of the water in the tub. Nevertheless, the recurrent wave "knows" where the center is. The center is the place where the wave disappears, or "goes out of the water."

An external trauma that enters the body, by contrast, creates a type of shock wave that causes an altered—probably an increased—wave pattern frequency at the entry place. The trauma may even have this effect at a distant area if it is strong enough.

The body is obliged to cope with the incoming wave pattern by integrating this incoming energy in a way that causes the least possible disturbance to the Tide and the midline function of the body. The final outcome, in most cases, is that the wave pattern becomes uncentered, and the tissues that are most intrinsically activated by the waves (eg, the fluid-containing tissues of the extracellular matrix, cerebrospinal fluid, and arteriolar/venous fields) progressively adapt to a slightly divergent pattern of exchange and interference. In addition, the intimate structure of the body reorganizes itself, eventually becoming fixed in an altered functional physiology.

Although a tissue or structure may retain in its memory (ie, its intrinsic organization) the old center of the long Tide, the disturbing pattern obliges the structure to function in an altered way. However, if the structure is provided with the proper support, it can find its way back to the midline feeling of the original wave pattern.

The traumatic symptom is the only landmark that indicates the Tide has been lost. But this symptom is also the body's "best friend," because it constitutes the means by which a good osteopath will be able to use its indicative value as a tool for reharmonizing the fluctuation of the Tide.

When one listens to the vital expression of the Tide, one should be particularly aware of slight deviations of the longitudinal pattern. For the osteopath, it is sufficient to guide the Tide in the aberrant direction to reintegrate the disturbed center into the longitudinal fluctuation. As W.G. Sutherland stated, a slight pressure upon the best-adapted site of the cranium usually suffices to reharmonise the Tide. In Sutherland's words, "Rely upon the Tide."

8.5 Balancing the body toward homeostatic functioning: the real power of healing

Homeostatic need is easily perceived when one studies intracellular exchange, cell-to-cell exchange, and cell-to-environment interaction. A certain electrolyte and ionic composition supports adaptive balancing in many kinds of cellular activities. It guarantees adaptability and restoration of original physiological values. This means that under normal, healthy conditions, the tissue and the cell are capable of leaving their original state to react and adapt, and to return toward their original state. Each cell possesses an inner balance by which it is capable of performing these processes.

The oxidation/reduction reactions and the subsequent changes in hydrogen ion concentration are expressions of the capability of the structure to achieve balance between safe barriers to inner and outer changes. On an electrolytic level, one could conceive of the electron as a keen expression of the capability of the cell to adapt to and express different states of physiology.

The whole structure of the body and its subsequent activities are expressions of either homeostatic or allostatic behaviors. A reactive body can balance between homeostasis and brief allostatic states. By this means, it is capable of restoring health.

Each cell possesses a biochemical and biomechanical pattern by which it serves its own referential framework and that of the whole structure. The balance is sustained by electron poising, by alkaline/hydrostatic ranges, by enzymatic shifts, by pivots in the vegetative nervous tonus, and by alterations in the immune-endocrine domain. This biochemical and bioelectrical system serves to construct and support structure—meaning that the structure should express the referential frame of the cell microenvironment.

Each cell possesses a spatial and structural organization consisting of a nucleus, cytoplasm, and membranes, linked by a cytoskeleton. This framework creates a balance to ensure survival of the cell. The cell not only depends upon biochemistry to survive, but it needs the cytoskeleton for transmission of power and for the creation of memory. Memory of the cell lies in the organization, orientation, and polarization of the microtubules in its interior.

Motion, motility, and contraction/expansion are expressions of the functioning of the mechanical transmission of chemical balancing. Mobility and motion are the most useful tools for the osteopath to evaluate the general condition of the body. However, the interpretation of a loss of mobility and motion should go beyond the mechanical expression of a change in the fields of exchange. It should be interpreted as an expression of history. Changes that have been expressed in the body at the tissue level indicate that the subtle fields of tissue exchange have been modified.

In osteopathy, we talk about the body as a balanced state of physiological interchange. In this balanced state, all tissues express the same quality of balanced interchange. W.G. Sutherland wrote about balanced membranous and ligamentous interchange as a quality present not only at the mechanical level, but also at the level of vital exchange. Getting in touch with the vital principle seemed to be the ultimate goal for Sutherland so that health could be restored.

R. Becker, as Sutherland's successor, was surely the most motivated person to propagate this idea about the art of healing. [13] The balance point and the still point are used as the royal pathway to reach the unattainable domain of dynamic interchange, the "drugstore" of the body in all its facets.

In my opinion, the aim of every osteopath should be to use all the physical indications of the body to discern as quickly as possible the unique level of energy disturbance of the body and to recover this loss. The loss is not focalized in a certain anatomical level. Instead, it belongs to the whole field of interaction of that particular level. It is also situated in specific space/time units that belong to the history/memory of the body.

It seems evident that loss of mobility and motion are useful indicators, but they only open the realm of subtle contact with the body that has been confined to tissue physiology. Tissue has to be studied in its metabolic, chemical, and physical properties before

8

we can communicate with it. And we need to reach as far as possible to touch the tissue's energetic field without losing ourselves in vague terminology of energetic interpretation.

Energy exchange is a state of equilibrated balanced interchange. One can feel it at the equilibriums in tension, direction, and density of tissue. This physiological state of balanced interchange opens the gateway to the intimate level of the body—to the story of the body contained in the stacked time/space units of its intimate memory.

The tissue level is the meeting place between the physiological needs of the body to "*move*" and the vital needs of the body to "*express*" life. It should be the place where the vital breath (including its generated wave patterns) meets the physical capacity of the body, to express this vital power as motion and mobility.

The real fulcrum [14] is the place where forces (ie, life forces of all kinds) meet, disappear, or reorganize. This fulcrum has to be reconsidered in osteopathic language, because it has been incorrectly thought of as a mechanical support for balancing the body. We need to understand that the fulcrum is the place where the body is enabled to work on its own health, with health meaning more than merely mechanical balance.

The fulcrum enables the body to harmonize on the physical, chemical, and electrical levels. This is the miracle of osteopathy—that it offers the right tool to the body for self-healing. The fulcrum offers freedom of time and space and supports the body's vital power to restore. This is something like the "meta-moment" described by H. Bergson.[4] [15]

Thus, the fulcrum could be the balance place between the physical capacities and the energetic factors determining the body's expression in life. Without the fulcrum, there is no motion; without motion, there is no expression of life.

REFERENCES
[1] Beloussov LV. The Dynamic Architecture of a Developing Mechanism. Dordrecht, Netherlands: Kluwer Academic Publishers, 1998.
[2] Blechschmidt E. Sein und Werden. Stuttgart, Germany: Verlag Urachhaus, 1982.
[3] Sills F. The embryological ordering principle. The Fulcrum. 1999;14:1–8.
[4] Sutherland WG. Teachings in the Science of Osteopathy. Cambridge, MA: Rudra Press, 1990:34,35,168.
[5] El-Khazen S. DNA: The gateway to time. NeuroQuantology. 2009;7:152–175.
[6] Becker RO, Selden G. The Body Electric: Electromagnetism And The Foundation Of Life. New York, NY: William Morrow, 1986.
[7] Hers HG. Science, non-science et fausse science. Paris, France: L'Harmattan, 1998:31–35.
[8] Poirier J, Ribadau Dumas J-L. Le système limbique. Paris, France: Laboratoires Hoechst, 1978:13–23.
[9] Rochedreux J. La mémorisation tissulaire, un vécu ostéopathique. 1995:22–25.
[10] Grey JA. The Psychology of Fear and Stress. New York, NY: McGraw-Hill, 1971:53–68.
[11] Sutherland WG. Contributions of Thought: The Collected Writings of William Garner Sutherland. 3rd ed. Portland, OR: Sutherland Cranial Teaching Foundation, 2002.
[12] Becker R. Life in Motion. Portland, OR: Stillness Press, 1997.
[13] Becker R. The Stillness of Life. Portland, OR: Stillness Press, 2000.
[14] Russell W. A New Concept of the Universe. Waynesboro, VI: University of Science and Philosophy, 1989.
[15] Bergson H. L'évolution créatrice. Paris, France: Felix Alcan, 1907.

---

4 [a]Bergson H. *Time and Free Will:* An Essay on the Immediate Data of Consciousness. London, United Kingdom: George Allen and Unwin, 1916.

CHAPTER

9 Mental image and its therapeutic value

9.1 Finding mind: the way to the mental image

The term "mental image" is evoked frequently as a useful unit in osteopathy. However, there is some confusion regarding its value in osteopathic treatment. For many osteopaths, mental image relates to a skill. For other osteopaths, mental image refers more often to a mystical level of perception than to any genuine awareness of the space/time expression offered by the patient.

An osteopath working with a mental image may appear to be using a subjective, nonscientific methodology in his or her approach to the patient. That is the reason we have tried to take a philosophical approach toward the meaning and intrinsic value of this concept.

Mental image as an osteopathic tool should probably be regarded as a final state of awareness resulting from the interference between the therapist and patient. This type of awareness is supported by the tools the therapist possesses, beginning with subjective guesses about the actual state of the patient. Sooner or later, the therapist is directed toward the subjective world of interference between mind and body. This relies upon deeper knowledge of the reciprocal exchange and interdependence between matter and energy, suggesting that there is no matter without a probability of exchange. Even the highest mountains—immovable and eternal in appearance—exist as matters of probability.

Likewise, the body may seem more or less constant in its appearance, but it is continuously changing, with exchanges between its inner and outer environment. It functions as a biological open system that depends upon thermodynamic laws.

One could ask what is really meant by the word "consciousness." Are there different types of consciousness? Is it an evident process that depends upon sheer sensorial exchange between matter and energy (ie, having a conscious perception of the object)? Or is it related to a well-ordered mental process that is capable of interfering with its own matter (ie, the self looking at itself).

Apparently, mind and matter are interdependent. When energy emanates from brain matter or interferes with it, mind appears as a kind of independent faculty of freedom that offers the possibility of creating a personalized form of perception, awareness, and cognition. We can conceive of mind as a form of positive entropy that results from a transformation of energy into a subtle state of awareness. Mind could be an interchangeable or a shared state of activity between two separated states of matter at the same moment (and, eventually, the same space).

Only when energy leaves the body at death does the question arise if mind is free or lost. Death could be conceived of as a final state of energy loss—definite entropy without a way back. Does the dying person experience it as a psychological process or as an ultimate physical awareness—a disintegration of physical sensations and feelings in our perceptual potential of the brain? This kind of awareness has not been well-defined, neither during the dying process nor during the living state.[1]

Dying is not so much a way of losing mind as it is a way of transitioning mind into non-relatedness. Energy that becomes unrelated to matter can eventually function as information if there is a receptor. Otherwise, one can only suppose that it becomes latent in an unidentified state.

Apparently consciousness and, related to it, the brain are more appropriate for storing information (structure) than for coping with energy loss (entropy).

---

[1] Curiously, dying is defined as a process and life as a state, even though one experiences life as process and death is a definite state.

In a certain way, the brain tries to minimize entropy (loss of energy) and to increase its possibilities for stability and storing information. [1]

We can propose that information is energy stored in an appropriate structure and referring to a certain order. We consider entropy as a loss of unfixed information. This is interesting because we all refer to our experiences by means of quanta or qualia. We never relate to pure life experience. H. Bergson defined this type of state as a metamoment. [2] Being without any form of reference seems to be an unknown state of existence.

What is the secret of the exchange between matter and energy, between body and mind? Are cognition and our evolutionary progression in consciousness a predisposed, pre-organized expression of an orchestrated program? Could it be that this program is precoded in the genome or in the frequencies of energy compounds that interact with the genetic code during a specific space/time schedule? [3]

The genome and the DNA strings could function as "probability units"[2] that are dependent for their activation upon a "photon trapping" process at a subtle level. [4, 5] This observation shifts our concept about origin to a more electrophysical level from a chemical-molecular level.

Can we conclude that our bodies are a kind of exchangeable energy, and that we all represent a certain passageway through the space/time units of life? In a certain sense, we are a mere physical expression of wave patterns that, through activation of specialized cells and tissues, represent a certain degree of referential interference with our inner and outer environment.

We probably create ourselves in the environment in which our evolution proceeds and progresses. We are the creator and the participant of our own environment, and of the story it contains.

The question arises if one can truly understand the transitional zone in which matter ends and mind surges. Should mind be defined as a cognitive and psychological unit, or should mind be considered as a physical process orchestrated by complex interactions between all the different body systems? These body systems and their fine-tuned interactions could be the carrier of subtle energy exchanges and phase-building that are necessary for creating mind processes. [6] "Mind expression" probably starts at the level of the transmembranous Ca^2-channel or the Na/K pump. It is not distillated only at the level of specialized interference between neuron clusters in the brain.

Is it possible to reduce the mind to a mere electrical/ionic process? Do we have to study the physics of mind, in which information is interpreted as quanta of electromagnetic energy converted into frequency/time scales, resulting in "log-ons" that express space/time units, such as memory and probability? [1] Is mind based on ionic/electromagnetic processes dependent upon refinement of integrative patterns, such as phase building, frequency patterns, and coherency?

Of course, mind cannot be considered as a physical unit only, though part of it can be studied in that way. We have to consider the origin of consciousness as a state of specialized awareness related to the inner and outer environment. Our anthropocentric concept of the universe has made the mind a property of human consciousness that seems able to orchestrate history and dominate nature and cosmology. A little arrogance and recklessness insidiously appear in this anthropocentrism.

Another question arises: When do we become conscious about ourselves? Do we need different selves to have gradients of consciousness, as described by A. Damasio? [7] Does mind relate to consciousness in the same way that thinking relates to mind?

Thinking and verbal communication seem to be the explicit tools of the evolutive mind. Mind functions as an expression of matter transformation that "dissipates" into quanta of frequency patterns, which can combine into flows of exchangeable information between appropriate forms of consciousness. Matter "contains" mind and appears as an intermediate between the energetic part of mind and the part we call consciousness. In a certain sense, this means that each form contains a part of mind constellated as a probability of information.

Hoffmann considered mind as residing inside each organ of the body, with each organ having its own mind (eg, liver mind, stomach mind, kidney mind). [8] It is worth considering the statement of Descartes, "cogito ergo sum" (In think, therefore I am), which we might convert into "sum ergo cogito" (I am, therefore I think). Damasio calls it the "brain-mind-body problem," because every kind of consciousness seems to depend upon a complex program—a web reflecting patterns built upon frequency coherency—the brain makes of the body. That means that mind is a part of body consciousness and depends upon information in the body consciousness.

During the earliest prenatal development, one can detect a protocognitive consciousness and, starting around the seventh month, a precognitive consciousness. The former represents a vague awareness of the body, revealed as automatic movements and sucking. These movements and consciousness do not seem to be linked to the cortex by the thalamic pathway. Rather, they appear to be concentrated at the level of the brain stem, which represents the first force plate of the information gathering of the central nervous system (CNS). The latter depends upon a more established network, with thalamocortical pathways and corticothalamic circuits.

As one can see, all these levels of consciousness maturation appear during precise stages of fetal and postnatal development and maturation (➤ Fig. 9.1). Furthermore, consciousness leading to cognition can be subdivided into subconscious, unconscious, and conscious levels of awareness. All of these stages are based on the first levels of consciousness arising during embryonic and fetal development. They function as referential microtimes that support the building of memory and cognition (➤ Fig. 9.2).

Apparently, mind matures into "the deep" of bodily development and bodily maturation during prenatal life. Consciousness appears in the physical world of awareness as a progression and summation of microstages of consciousness. These microstages are related to the progressive morphodynamic transformation of the embryonic body in its relation to an increasingly complex brain.

In its early stages, this process of microgenesis is related to the brain's awareness of body sensations that are meticulously stacked in different microtimes of brain staging—until the full brain landscape is built. Microtimes of consciousness are initially related to structuring processes of the brain. Over time, they become increasingly related to complex expressions of mind. [6] The energetic patterning and exchanges between different developmental fields become better organized, and the mind expresses an increased capability of broader interference with the outer and inner environment of consciousness and cognition.

It seems as if the development of mind relies upon the increasing possibilities of the body for storing and freeing energy. In a certain way, the development of the body seems supported by an increased amount of stored energy that modulates its progressive development. This information proceeds in a bottom-up direction to the brain and supports different phases of brain maturation, as displayed in the figure (➤ Fig. 9.2).

The body is like a linear database that provides essential information for acquiring more complex mind patterns. It functions as a flexible past that permits the actualized state to transform in more complex patterns or to find simplified and automatic solutions for adaptation. Mind is stacked in body processes, such as cellular and molecular information that, depending on the circumstances, is released as memory support for actuality.

Progressively, the body and mind become inseparable units that together represent the self (➤ Fig. 9.3). The body is the carrier of energy compounds that are offered to the brain in different quanta and qualia. When the right impulse elicits a coherency between body and brain, a spontaneous consciousness, related to that of corresponding lived space/time units, appears. Everything depends upon the right support, the right time, and the right place for

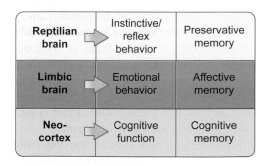

Fig. 9.1 P. McLean discerns three evolutionary phases in brain consciousness, each of them related to a particular faculty of consciousness.

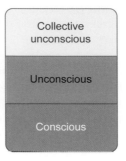

Reptilian brain	Instinctive behavior	Preservative memory
Limbic brain	Emotional behavior	Affective memory
Neo-cortex	Cognitive function	Cognitive memory

Collective unconscious
Unconscious
Conscious

Fig. 9.2 The different levels of consciousness related to the different states of mind, as proposed by A. Stevens

evoking or stacking information. The body refers to stacked information and offers the brain the possibility of an actualized state in the present or future. The body/brain unit waits for synchronization between impulse and frequency in the brain, leading to a time-related mind expression.

Mind is related to time because matter apparently evolves and resolves (or resumes) in time scales. Mind is a measure of time; it is not the master of time. It links the experiences and interpretations of time-separated events to a linear timescale. [9] The body appears as a database of separated timescales that, when activated appropriately, offers the possibility to the brain of evoking memorized bits of interference and using this information in current or future states of consciousness.

The brain evolved as an orchestra leader able to switch on and off the multiple space/time units stored by the body. The first step of its evolution was bottom-up. The more it contained complex patterns of activation, the more it started to build its own memory stacking at different levels of brain maturation. Eventually, the brain could compose its own "story" and impose it on the body. At that moment, it started to function top-down.

These two functions coincide with the two stages of embryonic/fetal maturation of the brain, in which the thalamocortical pathways develop first, followed by the corticothalamic pathways. The brain is able to store electrical energy patterns at specific receptivity for particular frequencies. When these frequencies are activated, the brain elaborates a specific action/memory pattern that is transmitted top-down to the body. These frequency patterns also permit the brain to have its proper level of experience interpretation evolve at the level of mind, independent of body/brain exchange.

The Referential Self

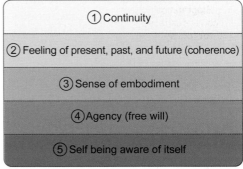

1 Continuity

2 Feeling of present, past, and future (coherence)

3 Sense of embodiment

4 Agency (free will)

5 Self being aware of itself

Fig. 9.3 The stepwise complexity of patterning of mind creates the possibility of an increasingly referential Self.

These mind experiences are increasingly related to the mechanisms of a personalized timescale that creates different forms of self-experience (➤ Fig. 9.4). It is as if during its genesis, the mind started to lead its own life in complex regions of the brain, and, in so doing, achieved the possibility for creating its own history. Mind started to control mind.

Still, mind remains bound to body, dependent upon the merging of relevant stages of body functions that have been stored in tissue memory during its development. These developmental peculiarities can reappear under certain stressful circumstances. They can be the motor for the uncontrollable power of emotions that either feed or disturb mind activity. The body interferes with the interactions between body/mind and brain/mind in such a way that it results in a process of suppression/activation that could activate or destabilize the compromise between mind/mind control.

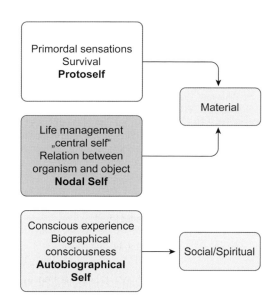

Fig. 9.4 A. Damasio distinguishes two different time scales corresponding to three types of Self.

The process of "thinking about the thinking" is partly dependent upon body awareness. That is precisely the level at which disease can start its neverending attempts at disrupting the balance between thought and feeling and between body function and mind control. Intuition is partly based upon stacked bodily memory; mind-thought is based upon the progressive experience of evolutive cognitive processes. Mind plays the role of an expansive dome upon physical processes, refining experience into increasingly complex patterns.

Mind is distilled in frequency patterns that rely upon body/mind and brain/mind interferences, which display common features for most people. That means that a mind is particularly sensitive to the frequencies displayed by other minds in their time and space experiences.

The power of a mind is not only its capability of thinking about thinking, but also its reliance upon the full history of body/mind interaction and this history's final integration into the cognitive domain. [7] By this means, the mind can even think about the thoughts of others and estimate their value or threat.

By synchronizing itself through frequency interferences, the mind is able to get in phase with other physical and mental neurological frequency trains

and to build a coherency field extending outside itself. This is probably the way in which mind can convert outside information into a representative mental image, which includes awareness of the therapist's own mind. This type of awareness ranges from bodily structure to emotional and cognitive contents.

The combination of all these feelings and sensations could result in a combined, focused realization of the actual state of the mind. This focusing is what the medical doctor does by interrogating the patient and exploring the anamnestic history of the patient. We are convinced that this is an art by which part of the diseased state is analyzed regarding causality. However, the real art of the medical doctor during treatment is to install a program that creates the tools for healing. This process relies upon the combination of intuition, experience, and knowledge of the therapist.

It could be that during the anamnesis and during the physical examination of the patient, a screening process takes place that does not completely rely upon the skills of the therapist. Rather, the therapist is able to use the accumulation of earlier integrated information gathered by different sources during medical practice. The experienced therapist can combine stored information with renewed knowledge, analyzing the unattended information. This process is not purely cognitive, but also intuitive. The common field between both is the place where the mental image appears and where it adds a supportive moment to treatment.

We can describe the mental image as the "third field" that progressively grows between the field of the therapist and that of the patient. It contains all of the information necessary for exchange and coherence between the two fields of interference. To the therapist, it relates to all of the knowledge necessary to understand the problem.[3]

If we accept the existence of a "third field"—the field between therapist and patient—it is possible that much of the analytical process occurs in a time scale that is faster than the normal latency times

---

[3] A. Chila translates the significance of the third field for osteopaths with the following group of questions: "Is there a lesion, where is the lesion, what is the lesion?"

9

needed for creating coherent thoughts. The brain is capable of creating a consciousness field at a time scale of 300 to 500 milliseconds—much faster than the conscious contents we communicate which each other. The third field is a precursor that gives potential to adaptation and participation of the patient and the therapist. In addition, it is able to relate and accommodate to the space/time schedules needed for efficient interference with the patient's problem. To the patient, it creates the feeling of empathy and the sensation of feeling secured by an outside person who knows about the problem.

These two understreams of consciousness—one from the patient and the other from the therapist—create the most favorable field for healing. All the tools needed for therapeutic practice will be automatically adapted at the particular space/time scale in which the problem must be treated. The healing point of treatment can be reduced to one specific locus, one specific cell, or one specific physical interference with the body.

REFERENCES

[1] Pribram KH. Brain and Perception: Holonomy and Structure in Figural Processing. New York, NY: Routledge, 2011.

[2] Bergson H. Time and Free Will: An Essay on the Immediate Data of Consciousness. New York, NY: George Allen & Unwin, 1916.

[3] El-Khazen S. DNA. The gateway to time. NeuroQuantology. 2009;7:152–175.

[4] Ho M-H. The Rainbow and the Worm: The Physics of Organisms. Singapore: World Scientific Publishing, 1998.

[5] Ho M-H, Popp F-A, Warnke U. Bioelectrodynamics and Biocommunication. Singapore: World Scientific Publishing, 1994.

[6] Bachmann T. Microgenetic Approach to the Conscious Mind. Philadelphia, PA: John Benjamins Publishing Company, 2000.

[7] Damasio A. L'autre moi-même. Paris, France: Odile Jacob, 2010.

[8] Hoffman H. Esoteric Osteopathy. Philadelphia, PA: Herbert Hoffman, 1906.

[9] Cheng F. The Way of Beauty: Five Meditations for Spiritual Transformation. Rochester, VT: Inner Traditions International, 2009.

Index